Who's Afraid of AAC?

CW01335237

AAC strikes fear into the hearts of professionals and families alike. Confusion, fear or denial often accompany a first encounter with AAC. AAC is weird, and complicated. Signs are confused with symbols, people have no idea how a switch can help someone talk, and the array of communication devices, software and apps is mind-boggling. Professionals often report feeling out of their depth.

Who's Afraid of AAC? The UK Guide to Augmentative and Alternative Communication is a new book which aims to demystify AAC. It will provide UK teachers and AAC professionals with an approachable guide to AAC and an easy-to-use toolkit of AAC ideas. The book covers the life span, from the first introduction of AAC with a baby or toddler, through Primary and Secondary School, on to University and into the working world, and changing circumstances with acquired conditions. We need to be ambitious: communication competency, literacy, academic and professional success and meaningful social participation are the goals. We need to negotiate the Hub and Spoke model and EHCPs on the way!

This resource aims to disseminate valuable research evidence, translating recommendations into best practice. There is advice on combining core and fringe vocabulary from Day 1, teaching phonics to a non-verbal student, writing meaningful EHCP outcomes and short-term targets, and relevant vocabulary for life stages. This is a book that practitioners will dip into and out of for years to come.

Alison Battye is a practising speech and language therapist who specialises in children with Complex Needs and Autism Spectrum Disorder. She has worked across mainstream and special school settings from Foundation Stage to Further Education, supporting practitioners in implementing AAC with children and young people.

Who's Afraid *of* AAC?

The UK Guide to Augmentative and Alternative Communication

Alison Battye

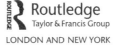

Routledge
Taylor & Francis Group

LONDON AND NEW YORK

First published 2018
by Routledge
2 Park Square, Milton Park, Abingdon, Oxon OX14 4RN

and by Routledge
711 Third Avenue, New York, NY 10017

Routledge is an imprint of the Taylor & Francis Group, an informa business

British Library Cataloguing-in-Publication Data
A catalogue record for this book is available from the British Library

Library of Congress Cataloging-in-Publication Data
A catalog record has been requested

ISBN: 978-1-911186-17-5 (pbk)
ISBN: 978-1-315-17291-0 (ebk)

Typeset in Meta
by Apex CoVantage, LLC
Printed by Ashford Colour Press Ltd

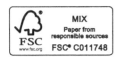

Contents

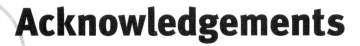

Acknowledgements

This book would not have been possible without the expertise and support of my colleagues at the Kent and Medway Communication and Assistive Technology (KM CAT) Service. This team is an inspiration. Special thanks go to:

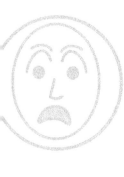

Heather Bovingdon, Friedl Jansen van Vuuren, Freya Senior, Ruth Coenen, Fiona Panthi and Maria Touliatou for their proof-reading on communication, language acquisition and no-tech, low-tech and light-tech AAC.

Debbie Bailey, Penny Harman, Karen Al Khina, Jodie Rogers and Julie Bradford for their proof-reading on access and mounting.

Amy Williams, Claire Ottaway, Sarah Ayres, Tina Harrison and Rachel Dormedy for their wealth of practical AAC expertise which has informed every chapter in the book, with particular thanks for the content of *Shared Voices*. Thank you especially to Amy, who has taught me so much about Aided Language Stimulation in the classroom.

Nicole Tumber, Hester Mackay, Laura Kilvington-Smith, Christine Cotterill, Claire Riches and Terri Rutherford for advising on literacy and curriculum resources.

Rachel Keen for guidance on EHCPs.

Nana Odom for her unrivalled knowledge of software packages.

Sarah Lloyd-Cocks and Ladan Najafi for being supportive of this project.

Hilary Gardner at Communication Matters for her extreme efficiency and ability to find relevant information fast. Bronagh Blaney for information on AAC in Northern Ireland.

Katharine Buckley, Claire Latham, Will Wade, Amy Follows, Ian Foulger, Hannah Church, Trevor Mobbs, Siobhan Bhutel, John Bullock, Hannah Fitzpatrick, Chris Thornton, Cara Hubers, Sarah Beyl, Mick Davies, Emily Webb, Peter Butler and Ben Johnston for their support in sharing their fantastic AAC resources.

Katherine Coe for her pieces of written work used in Chapter 12, and Amy Clark for her incredible piece of creative writing used in Chapter 8. You are inspirational young women.

Special thanks also go to:

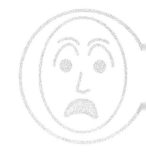

> Catherine Thomas, Wendy Coggins and Wendy Callaghan, my SLT godmothers.
>
> My daughter, Caty Weeks, for her advice about street-talk and social identity in Secondary School.
>
> My daughter, Amelie Weeks, for her thoughts on social inclusion in Primary School.
>
> My step-daughter, Kitty Dodds, for her thoughts on the front cover.
>
> My step-son, William Dodds, for the loan of his spinny chair.
>
> My partner, Stephen Dodds, for reminding me to eat and drink.
>
> My parents, Jan and Phil Battye, for instilling the message "yes, we can!"

Thanks to Widgit Symbols for their permission for the symbols on the cover and throughout the book: Widgit Symbols © Widgit Software 2002–2017.

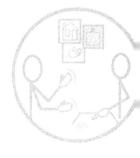

Abbreviations

AAC	Augmentative and Alternative Communication
ABA	Applied Behavioural Analysis
ALS	Amyotrophic Lateral Sclerosis
ASC	Autism Spectrum Condition
ASD	Autism Spectrum Disorder
AT	assistive technology
BATA	British Assistive Technology Association
BSL	British Sign Language
BVPS	British Picture Vocabulary Scales
CAMHS	Child and Adolescent Mental Health Services
CARLA	Computer-Based Accessible Receptive Language Assessment
CAT	Communication and Assistive Technology
CELF-5	Clinical Evaluation of Language Fundamentals
CP	Cerebral Palsy
CVC	consonant-vowel-consonant
CYP	child/young person
DLA	Disabled Living Allowance
DSA	Disability Students' Allowance
DVD	Developmental Verbal Dyspraxia
EFA	Education Funding Agency
EHCP	Education, Health and Care Plan
EKOS	East Kent Outcomes System
EMG	electromyographic
EYFSP	Early Years Foundation Stage Profile
FE	further education
GP	general practitioner
ISAAC	International Society for Augmentative and Alternative Communication
JCQ	Joint Council for Qualifications
LAMP	Language Acquisition through Motor Planning
MND	Motor Neurone Disease
MS	Multiple Sclerosis
MSA	Multiple Systems Atrophy
NLG	Natural Language Generation
NRA	Non-verbal Reading Approach
NSPCC	National Society for the Prevention of Cruelty to Children
OT	Occupational Therapist
PALPA	Psycholinguistic Assessments of Language Processing in Aphasia

PCS   Picture Communication Symbols
PECS   Picture Exchange Communication System
PMLD   Profound Multiple Learning Disability
PODD   Pragmatic Organisation Dynamic Display
PSP   Progressive Supranuclear Palsy
RCSLT   Royal College of Speech and Language Therapists
RFID   radio frequency identification
SCBU   Special Care Baby Unit
SCRUFFY   Student-led, Creative, Relevant, Unspecified, Fun For Youngsters
SEN   Special Educational Need
SENCO   Special Educational Needs Coordinator
SEND   Special Educational Needs or Disabilities
SGD   Speech Generating Device
SLI   Specific Language Impairment
SLT   Speech and Language Therapist
SMART   Specific, Measurable, Achievable, Realistic, Time-Limited
SPAG   spelling, punctuation and grammar
SQA   Scottish Qualifications Authority
TA   Teaching Assistant
TAP   Therapy Assistant Practitioner
TBI   traumatic brain injury
TROG-2   Test for Reception of Grammar
VOCA   Voice Output Communication Aid
WLS   Widgit Literacy Symbols

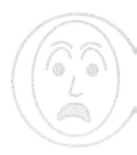

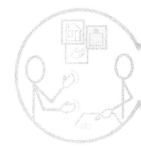

Chapter 1

What is communication?

Communication is the sharing of a message between two people.

One person sends a message, the other person receives it. There has to be a shared understanding of what the message means. There has to be an accepted mode of communication.

Only 7% of human communication is verbal. That is, only 7% is made up of spoken words organised into phrases or sentences. The other 93% is non-verbal.[1] Non-verbal communication may include body posture and gesture, facial expression and eye-pointing, or tone of voice and emphasis. The *way* we say something may completely change the meaning of the words and phrases we use.

Intentional and pre-intentional communication

Intentional communication is where the sender of the message consciously sends it to another person. They have the expectation that the receiver will try to interpret the message and act upon it.

Pre-intentional communication is a developmental stage where the sender of the message has not realised that they can consciously send a message to another person. A very young baby cannot help communicating a message that they are hungry, tired or in pain. As the baby gets older they learn that their caregiver is responsive to their unintentional communication. When the baby cries, they receive comfort. When they squeal in pleasure, the caregiver tickles them again. Gradually the baby's communication becomes *intentional*. They may "shout" to get attention. They may hold their arms out to be picked up. They may reach for a toy and look at their caregiver to request their help.

For a baby, child or even an adult to move from pre-intentional to intentional communication, they need a responsive adult to help them to make the leap. They need their caregiver to observe what they are looking at, listening to and to guess at what they are feeling and thinking. They need this responsive partner to recognise when they have misinterpreted a message, and to try again.

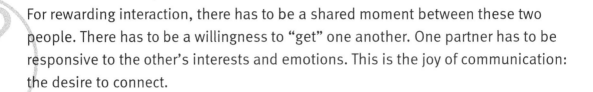

For rewarding interaction, there has to be a shared moment between these two people. There has to be a willingness to "get" one another. One partner has to be responsive to the other's interests and emotions. This is the joy of communication: the desire to connect.

The leap from pre-intentional to intentional communication usually happens near the end of the first year, but for some children with developmental delay, it may take longer. Some adults with profound learning difficulties may not have moved on from the pre-intentional stage. This is not to say that there is no communication, but that the responsive adult has to adapt their communication to interpret the message sensitively. *Intensive Interaction*[2] is a therapeutic approach for pre-intentional communicators and can help to move them on to intentional communication.

Multi-modal communication

We are all *multi-modal* communicators. We do not communicate using speech alone.

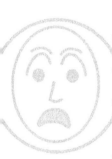

We supplement our spoken words with:

- Body language (proximity, turning towards or away, being relaxed or tense);
- Eye contact (this can feel comfortable or it can feel too intense or avoidant);
- Eye-pointing (we look at something of interest, then at the person for a reaction);
- Facial expressions (e.g. widening our eyes to express interest, rolling our eyes to express annoyance);
- Pointing (e.g. when ordering in a café, when giving directions);
- Gesture (e.g. shrugging shoulders, beckoning or dismissing with our hands);
- Nodding or shaking our head;
- Noises (e.g. tutting, squealing, yelping, laughing, snorting);
- The loudness of our voice (e.g. this might suggest authority or secrecy);
- The rate at which we speak (e.g. we might speak more slowly for emphasis);
- The musicality of our tone (we are more tuneful with small children and when we want to keep someone's attention).

We use different types of verbal and non-verbal communication for different communication situations. At work we will tend to be more careful about what we say and do, and we are more guarded about what we reveal through our non-verbal communication. We wouldn't tend to pull a face of annoyance behind a colleague's back, or use a rude gesture. We would be more likely to use formal vocabulary and correct grammar. At home and in informal social situations, we are likely to be more relaxed, spontaneous and expressive with our non-verbal and verbal communication. We will use a slightly different vocabulary, including more colloquialisms and words that are associated with our cultural group. Our grammar may diverge from standard English. We might not need to finish our sentences because our intimate family and friends know what we mean. We might be louder, faster or more animated in these situations. These differences in communication style, which depend on the who, what, where, why and how we are communicating, are known as different *registers*.

What is language?

Language is a formalised system of communicating.

It is made up of a *vocabulary* of words, or signs, or symbols. Each word, sign or symbol carries a distinct meaning. Vocabulary can be organised into categories for meaning (e.g. animals vs. transport). Words can be related to one another according to different aspects of the word's meaning. For example, the word "dog" is related in different ways to the words "cat", "puppy", "pet", "fur", "wagging" and "wet". *Semantics* is the study of the meanings of words and how they relate to one another.

We can combine these words, signs or symbols in specific ways to this language. Each language has a set of rules about word order that cannot be broken. This is *syntax* or *grammar*. It includes rules about how some words can have different functions, like nouns, verbs and adjectives. Syntax determines what form a word can take. For example in English, nouns take on an "-s" ending to indicate there is more than one. Verbs can take on different endings; for example, in the present tense we add "-ing" to regular verbs.

We communicate for different reasons. These reasons are often referred to as the *functions of language*. They might also be referred to as *communicative functions*, because you do not always need language for them; you can use non-verbal communication. A few of these communicative functions are:

- To get someone's attention
- To request an item or an action
- To reject an item or an action
- To draw attention to something that is happening

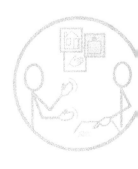

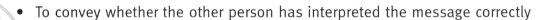

- To convey whether the other person has interpreted the message correctly
- To say something about an item or an action
- To comment on what is happening
- To check the other person's reaction to what is happening
- To ask a question
- To answer a question
- To tell a story
- To joke
- To explain what you are thinking
- To explain what you are feeling.

In this list, the early functions can be carried out without a formalised language, but it is hard to move through the list beyond the fifth item, without some form of language. This aspect of language is called the social use of language, or the *pragmatics* of language.

How do communication and language fit together?

Communication is wider than language. Communication includes non-verbal communication. It includes the use of signs and symbols. It can also include a formalised language, which is usually verbal.

There are languages consisting of manual signs, not spoken words, as in British Sign Language (BSL). British Sign Language is not related to English in any way. It is a distinct language, with different rules for vocabulary and grammar.

For the purposes of this book, we will tend to focus on *signing systems*, not sign language.

Makaton[3] and Signalong[4] are signing systems, but they are not languages in their own right. They are mapped onto the local language, which in the UK is usually English. They are accompanied by spoken language. They support the spoken language, but cannot be used independently of it. You always speak as you sign with Makaton or Signalong.

Symbol sets such as Widgit Literacy Symbols (WLS) and Picture Communication Symbols (PCS) also support spoken language. In the UK, they are used to support spoken English.

Multi-modal communication to suit the situation

Multi-modal communication encompasses all of these modes of communication: non-verbal communication, spoken language, and signs and symbols. We are all multi-modal communicators. This is what makes us resourceful, successful communicators in a number of different communication situations and environments. Some situations lend themselves to spoken communication, for example, debating a political issue. Some situations lend themselves to non-verbal communication, for example, giving a subtle message to a partner across a room. Most situations involve a mixture of modes. If one mode fails, we will bring in another. We learn how to employ different strategies as we become competent communicators.

What is empathic interaction?

Empathic interaction is the sense that another person really gets you. They have picked up on your mood, the feelings behind your words, gestures, facial expressions. They are intuitively responding to your emotional needs. It can give a sense of joy to both partners.

Of course we don't always achieve this! It is a special magic that happens sometimes, with some people. But it is what gives us a sense of wellbeing and connection with other people.

We don't need words to achieve empathic interaction. Can you remember a time when you had a non-verbal exchange with a complete stranger because you both noticed something and felt the same thing about it? You may have exchanged a knowing grin, or a look of mutual shock. We can also achieve this with children and adults who have very limited communication. Just by noticing their reaction to an event, and responding empathically can provide a moment of special connection for both of you.

We should always be aiming for empathic interaction. It doesn't have to be a happy moment. You could be sharing a moment of despair, frustration or rage. Being attuned to another person is incredibly important to both people's sense of wellbeing and connection.

What is AAC?

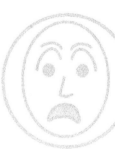

Augmentative and Alternative Communication (AAC) is any form of language or communication that is used to augment, or supplement, spoken language, or is used as an alternative to spoken language. There are many different types of AAC to meet the very different communication needs of the users. Some people may need AAC to support their understanding and expression. Some people may have very

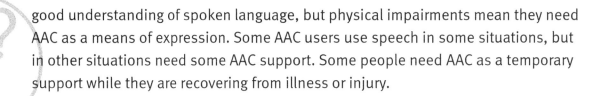

good understanding of spoken language, but physical impairments mean they need AAC as a means of expression. Some AAC users use speech in some situations, but in other situations need some AAC support. Some people need AAC as a temporary support while they are recovering from illness or injury.

AAC can be no-tech, in the case of signing. No special equipment is needed for no-tech. AAC can be low-tech, which usually means it is paper-based. This could be photos, pictures or symbols. It could be a symbol-based communication chart, or an alphabet chart. It could be a communication book. AAC can be light-tech. This will be a battery-operated device with recorded voice output. It may be single-message, multi-message, or have multiple paper overlays. High-tech AAC is a computer or tablet device, with a dynamic screen display, with digitised or synthesised voice output.

What is assistive technology?

Assistive technology, or AT, is any piece of equipment that has been made or modified to improve the functional capabilities of an individual with a disability. Assistive technology for people with physical impairments includes wheelchairs and walkers. Assistive technology for people with sensory impairments includes hearing aids or screen readers. It includes environmental controls, whereby an individual can control the heating, lighting or media in their home. It includes software to make learning or social media accessible. Some people will need AAC but not AT, for example, people with Autism Spectrum Condition. Some people will need AT but not AAC, for example, a person with Muscular Dystrophy who is able to speak. Some people need both, for example a person with four-limb Cerebral Palsy, or Motor Neurone Disease.

Access to AAC and AT

Access in this book is used to mean the way the individual accesses their AAC or AT. They may be able to use direct access: that is to point to a symbol or press a button. They may use indirect access, like switch-scanning. The same access solutions may be used for AAC and AT. For example, a young person may use eye-gaze technology for their communication package, for recording their work in school, and for controlling the TV and sending email at home. We need to provide holistic intervention for individuals, so that we are thinking about how they access their living space, wider community, education, work and the social world.

How many people need AAC?

It is estimated that 0.5% of the population could benefit from some type of AAC (1 in 200). 0.05% could benefit from high-tech AAC (1 in 2000).[5] This includes children and adults with developmental conditions such as Cerebral Palsy, Down

Syndrome, learning disabilities and Autism Spectrum Condition. Those with Specific Language Impairment and Developmental Verbal Dyspraxia also benefit from AAC. These children are not included in the figures. It is estimated that the prevalence of Specific Language Impairment is 5%.[6] There are also acquired conditions such as stroke and traumatic brain injury. Finally there are individuals with degenerative conditions such as Muscular Dystrophy in children, and Motor Neurone Disease, Multiple Sclerosis and Alzheimer's Disease in adults. The AAC-using population is therefore incredibly diverse, and individuals will have very different profiles of ability and need.

In the next chapter, we will look at how children typically acquire communication and language skills. This will inform the implementation of AAC for atypical language acquisition.

Notes

1 Mehrabian, A. (1972) *Silent Messages: Implicit Communication of Emotions and Attitudes*. Belmont, CA: Wadsworth.
2 Hewett, D., Barber, M., Firth, G. and Harrison, T. (2011) *The Intensive Interaction Handbook*. London: Sage.
3 http://makaton.org.
4 http://signalong.org.uk.
5 Communication Matters (2013) *Shining a Light on Augmentative and Alternative Communication*. Communication Matters Research Matters: An AAC Evidence Base Research Project – Final Report, on http://communicationmatters.org.uk
6 Law, J., Boyle, J., Harris, F., Harkness, A. and Nye, C. (2000) Prevalence and natural history of primary speech and language delay: Findings from a systematic review of the literature. *International Journal of Language and Communication Disorders*, 3(2), 165–188.

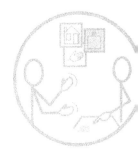

Chapter 2

Typical language development

The language development pyramid

The language development pyramid[1] is a helpful model for showing the component skills for language development. If you set about building a pyramid, you have to begin building at the bottom.

Attention and listening is the foundation for *play*. A baby needs to play to learn about the world around them, in order to start to *understand* language. They need to understand language in order to use it, that is, to start *talking*. They need to talk well before accurate speech sounds can be achieved.

One level is not complete before the next level begins to develop: they are developing concurrently, but the attainment at each level is dependent on the levels below.

I will now explain in more detail each level of the pyramid.[2]

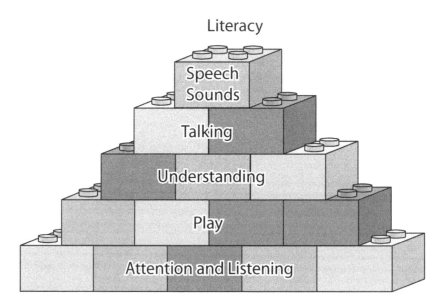

Adapted from The Communication Trust.

Diagram 2.1 Language development pyramid

Attention and listening

As soon as a baby is born (and in fact before this, in utero), they are able to distinguish between a human voice and other sounds. They show recognition of their caregivers' voices. A newborn baby is able to focus on a caregiver's face when they are being held, and shows a preference for looking at faces over other objects. Babies are soothed by gentle touch, and being held by a caregiver.[3] Babies are hard-wired to tune in to communication.

In the first year, caregivers spend a lot of time fine-tuning these attention and listening skills. The caregiver is responsive to everything the baby does. Unconsciously, we mirror the baby's facial expressions and echo their noises. This is *reciprocity*. We show the baby that they are not alone. We are noticing them, and we are trying to understand them.

The caregiver treats the baby as the most fascinating thing in the room, and everything the baby does is interpreted as meaningful and valid. For example, "oh, you have a tummy-ache!", "you like that song".

The baby has "mirror neurones" in their developing brain, which are activated by this type of interaction. This allows the baby to develop an understanding of their own and others' emotions.[4]

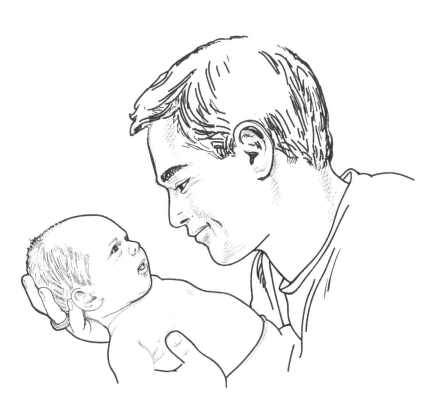

From early in a baby's life, we engage in *joint-attention*. Whatever they notice, we also notice. If they startle to a sound, we acknowledge the sound. If they peer at a cot mobile, or turn to look as someone enters the room, we also look. We may well do or say something to interpret this event. We reassure a startled baby by making soothing noises. We point at the cot mobile and make a delighted noise. We turn and wave at the person coming into the room. Gradually the baby learns *joint-referencing*. When something interesting or new happens, they look to their caregiver to gauge their response. They start to interpret the world through the social responses of others.

Every time a baby is being changed, getting ready to be fed, standing in their cot after a nap, or sitting up in their pram or rocker . . . the caregiver will always take the opportunity to make eye contact and will respond with *Parentese*, or *Infant-Directed Speech*.[5] They will use an interesting, more sing-song voice, they will emphasise and repeat important words, they will exaggerate their facial expressions and they will show the baby what they are talking about.

The baby learns to coordinate their looking and their listening skills. If they are face-to-face with a caregiver, they can see that their facial expressions and lip movements are consistent with the noises they are making. Looking and listening need to be coordinated when attending to someone else's communication.

At first, a baby will shift their gaze from a toy to a caregiver in order to hear what the caregiver is saying. Over time, the toddler will be able to take in what an adult is saying without the need for shifting their gaze. Listening becomes less effortful and more automatic.

When a toddler is playing with a toy and checking that the caregiver is also looking at the toy, the toddler starts to understand that the caregiver is talking about this toy. This is important for language growth. The toddler starts to assume that the adult is providing them with the relevant language for the situation.

Social communication skills, which include the use of empathic and reciprocal facial expressions, body language and tone of voice, develop concurrently alongside attention and listening. Caregivers spend a good year modelling these skills, every day, throughout the day.

Play

"Play" is a baby's way of exploring the world around them. They do this through their senses, mainly sight, sound and touch, and with their body movements.

A baby does not experience the world in the way an adult does. Though their eyes and ears may be fully functional, their brains have to learn how to interpret these sensory signals. They have to coordinate information from a number of different senses, to create a coherent experience of the world. When someone claps, we actually hear the clap after we see it. The brain interprets the signals as being simultaneous, because otherwise our experience of the world would be confusing and incoherent.

Babies' brains are changing enormously in the first year. As patterns of experience emerge, neural connections are made.

When experiencing a "ball", the baby will be exposed to the following: this object can be rolled, it feels smooth and cold in my mouth, it is hard to keep hold of, it is brightly coloured and spotty, it makes a jingly sound when I shake it. This involves different areas of the brain for tactile, visual and auditory information. It also involves proprioceptive, vestibular and motor patterns for sitting in this position, balancing, holding the ball, and shaking it up and down. Different parts of the brain become linked up like a road map. Some roads will not be used and will disappear. Some roads will become motorways because they are used all the time.

"Play" is sensorimotor in the first year. It is involves incoming sensory information, and outgoing motor movement from the baby.

There is also social play, with turn-taking games like "peekaboo" and rolling a ball to one another. Singing songs together, particularly those with fun actions, like "Round and Round the Garden" or "This Little Piggy," foster early turn-taking and joint-attention for play and for language-learning.

In the second year, pretend-play starts to develop. This begins as simple mimicry: the baby pretends to drink from a cup because this is what they have seen adults do. They get a positive response, so they are likely to do this again. As they learn about more objects and actions in their world, they build more diverse and more complex patterns of pretend-play.

Pretend-play is important for language development, because the baby has made an important cognitive link: the play cup stands for the real cup. It is a symbol. Words are also symbols. The word, sign or symbol "cup" stands for the real cup. This allows us to communicate about "cup" when it is not actually there.

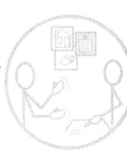

Understanding (receptive language)

In the later end of the first year, babies are learning about *cause-and-effect*. They are learning to anticipate what will happen if they carry out a particular action. For example, "if I squeal, then mum will look. If I drop this cup, it makes a loud noise on the floor. If I press this button, music plays". This predictability is very important for language development. The baby has learnt that there are patterns; there is order.

Towards the end of the first year, the baby can make some predictions about the world. Because every time they cry or shout or exclaim it has an effect on the adults around them, they will start to do these things with *communicative intent*. The baby understands that what they do is important, and that it communicates a message. Sometimes that message is misinterpreted, but that is OK, because most of the time it is correctly interpreted, and when it isn't, then at least they can see their caregiver is trying.

This is the very important shift from *pre-intentional* to *intentional communication*.

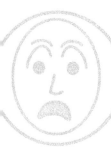

The baby starts to see that just as there are patterns in sensorimotor information (e.g. the cup always makes a sound when it is dropped on the kitchen floor), there are also patterns in what the adult does. The adult always says "uh-oh!" when something goes wrong. They always say "up" when they pick the baby up. They always say "bye bye" when someone leaves the room. This may also be accompanied by a particular gesture, facial expression or intonation pattern. The baby starts to build a collection of words that are understood. These may be "daddy", "dog" or "car". They will be personal to that baby's everyday life, and will be things or events that happen frequently and consistently. The child will learn that while they may look and feel slightly different, a beach ball and a tennis ball are both still "ball".

Social words and nouns (names for people, objects and places) tend to be easily learnt, as the adult can label them repeatedly, and there are usually lots of opportunities for modelling these words.

Verbs can more tricky to label at exactly the right time. You have to catch something as it "fell down" and label it at the right point. More general verbs like "gone" can be learnt fairly early. The more specific verbs tend to follow on when lots of nouns have been learnt.

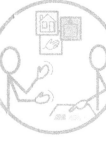

Adjectives will come later after repeated exposure specific situations. The more salient concepts like "hot", "wet" and "dirty" will be learnt before the less obvious experiences of "cold", "dry" and "clean".

Adults have to input language before the child can output language (input before output). A child may echo back a word without understanding it, but for them to use it with meaning, the child needs to first understand the word.

Talking (expressive language)

Sooner or later, if there are no sensory or motor difficulties, and no social communication difficulties, most babies will have a go at copying the communication behaviours of the adults. This will include talking. Their first attempts may be poorly executed, but that doesn't matter, because the adult is delighted, and makes a big fuss, and copies back what the baby just did, and so the baby is motivated to do it again.

There will be a few mistakes. For a while, all men are "daddy". All animals are "doggy". But the adults are supportive, and will say "yes, cat!" and so the child will understand the difference, even if they can't say it yet. Early on in expressive language development a few words may be used for a number of different phenomena.

The toddler soon learns that if they point to something and vocalise with rising intonation, their caregiver will give them the word for it.

This is a huge step. The child starts to lead their own language-learning. They just have to show the adults around them what they are interested in, and the adult supplies the right language at the right level.

The first few words tend to be acquired very slowly. However, like most skills, the brain learns how to learn the skill, and gets better and faster as it goes along. So a child may say three words at 15 months, 20 words at 18 months, 50 words at 2 years, and 200 words at 3 years. These are a minimum: many children will acquire words even faster, and will have 10 times as many words by 3 years.

Children with typically developing language can learn some words with just one exposure,[6] because they use all their other communication and language skills to quickly assess its meaning and learn its structure. They use the semantic and syntactic context of the words around it to work out what the word means and how it can be used in a sentence, and they use their phonological knowledge to remember its sounds.

Children begin by using single words, or phrases that are learnt whole, like "all gone".[7] When they have about 50 words in their expressive vocabulary, they start

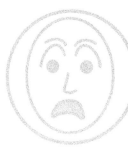

the creative process of combining words to make novel phrases. This typically starts by the time the child is 2 years old. Phrases are "telegraphic" at first: words will be combined without any grammatical inflections. Examples of early word combinations are "mummy sock" and "daddy gone". A range of meanings can be achieved through supplementing the verbal message with non-verbal communication, like tone of voice, and gesture.

Phrases become more complex over the next two years, and grammar starts to develop, so that children add the "little words" such as pronouns, prepositions, conjunctions and verb endings. They will over-generalise some rules, for example, irregular verb-endings or irregular plurals will still be confused (e.g. "I goed", "sheeps").

Adults tend to model language that is one step ahead of what the child can say.[8] So if a child isn't saying words yet, the adult will give a single word, and maybe show the thing they mean. Adults naturally and instinctively repeat what the child has said, and make it a little bit more sophisticated. For example if the child says "bird", the adult might say "the bird's *flying*", or "it's a *big* bird". They will highlight the new word by placing emphasis on it in the sentence. They will be delighted if the child says the new word or phrase back to them, and so the child will get social reinforcement.

Speech sounds (pronunciation)

If there has been no disruption to the child's visual or auditory input, they will make good approximations of the words modelled by adults. Adults will be intuitively familiar with simplifications the young child makes, and will repeat the word back clearly, so that even though the child can't say the word correctly yet, they will have an internal representation of how it should sound.

Speech sounds may get worse before they get better. At two to three-and-a-half, there will be a language explosion in the child, where they are learning vocabulary at such a fast rate, and starting to use longer phrases and sentences, and if something is going to give, it will tend to be speech sounds. However, most children will be able to store how the word should sound, and will use this to fine-tune their pronunciation when the production of language is becoming more automatic.

Social communication

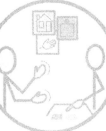

Social communication skills are diverse, and suffuse every aspect of non-verbal communication and spoken language. If I had to add them to the Language Development Pyramid, then they would be the cement that sticks the blocks together, to create coherence and shared meaning. Social communication skills include:[9]

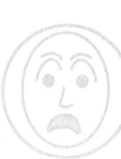

- The understanding and use of eye contact to engage and maintain another person's attention, and to show that we are engaged.

- The understanding and use of facial expressions, gestures and body language; reciprocity of these to show empathy and understanding.

- The understanding and use of body contacts and proximity, and the loudness and tone of voice, to modulate meaning and to show reciprocity and attunement.

- Topic maintenance and semantic contingency: responding to what the other person has said, and adding to this.

- Modulating what we say and how we say it; adjusting our style and content to our communication partner's needs and point of view.

- Adjusting our communication to suit the social context: depending on who we are talking to, where, what we are trying to convey, and why.

- Repairing communication breakdowns: clarifying the message if it has been misinterpreted; using different modes of communication as necessary.

Social communication skills continue to develop and become more refined throughout childhood and into adolescence. Understanding that what is in someone else's head is not the same as what is in ours, or *Theory of Mind*,[10] starts to develop from around four years of age, and this is important for attuning to the needs of others.

Spoken language competency

By 5 years old, the language development pyramid is more or less complete. Most children have achieved *spoken language competency*. They have acquired a wide-ranging vocabulary and understand word meanings (semantics). They know how to put words together into phrases and sentences, with words in the right order, and they are starting to use word endings and little words like "to" and "in" (grammar and syntax). They can pick up on subtleties of meaning from non-verbal communication and social context (pragmatics and social communication). They can even start to manipulate sounds in words, and to understand that words can be broken down into syllables and phonemes (phonology).

Written language (literacy)

Children become aware that language can be represented in print as they engage in shared reading with an adult. They start to realise that print carries meaning,

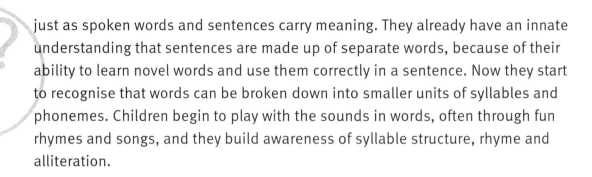

just as spoken words and sentences carry meaning. They already have an innate understanding that sentences are made up of separate words, because of their ability to learn novel words and use them correctly in a sentence. Now they start to recognise that words can be broken down into smaller units of syllables and phonemes. Children begin to play with the sounds in words, often through fun rhymes and songs, and they build awareness of syllable structure, rhyme and alliteration.

The "internal representation" of how a word should sound is vital for literacy development. The child will know that "dog" is quite distinct from "log" or "dig". The child may be able to say the first sound in a word, and learn that this sound has a particular visual representation, which looks like "d".

All children should be given the opportunity to move on from spoken language to written language. We will come back to this in Chapter 11.

Bilingual and multilingual language development

Children who are learning more than one language simultaneously from birth go through the same stages in language development. There may be a slight delay, but they will soon catch up with their monolingual peers. The benefits of bilingualism include better attention and listening, greater creativity and problem-solving.[11] There may be a period of "code-switching" whereby children sometimes mix languages.

Parents are advised to use their own mother tongue, or first language, with their child, so that they provide a good language model. If parents have different first languages, they should use their own first language with the child. Children quickly learn to associate a person with a language, and will only use that language with those they know speak it.

Once children have acquired one language, they tend to acquire a second fairly easily. Therefore it is not necessary to try to expose a child from birth to the dominant language in the country they live in. Children will not learn a second language from the TV or apps. They need a responsive communication partner who is proficient in the language.

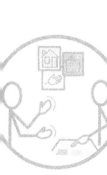

If no one at home speaks the dominant language of the country the child lives in, there is no need to artificially introduce it into the home. Children tend to acquire the dominant language easily once they attend nursery or school.

This chapter has focused on typical language development. In the next two chapters, we will consider atypical language acquisition.

Notes

1 This pyramid model has been used for many years by Speech and Language Therapists, with minor variations. This version is adapted from the Communication Trust in their online guidance *Communicating the Curriculum*. See http://communicationtrust.org.uk.

2 See *Stages of Speech and Language Development* on http://talkingpoint.org.uk for a useful poster showing ages and stages of language development.

3 Gerhardt, S. (2004) *Why Love Matters: How Affection Shapes a Baby's Brain*. London: Routledge, p. 23.

4 Ibid.

5 Snow, C. and Ferguson, C. (1979) *Talking to Children: Language Input and Acquisition*. Cambridge: Cambridge University Press.

6 Swingley, D. (2010) Fast mapping and slow mapping in children's word learning. *Language, Learning and Development*, 6(3), 179–183.

7 See Brown, R. (2013) *A First Language: The Early Stages*. Cambridge, MA: Harvard University Press, for detailed descriptions of early expressive language.

8 This is Vygotsky's "Zone of Proximal Development". Adults instinctively provide children with learning opportunities that are just inside their reach: not to easy and not too difficult. See Vygotsky, L. (1978) *Mind in Society: The Development of Higher Psychological Processes*. Cambridge, MA: Harvard University Press.

9 Dave Hewitt calls these "The Fundamentals of Communication" in Intensive Interaction. See http://intensiveinteraction.co.uk.

10 Baron-Cohen, S. (1997) *Mindblindness: An Essay on Autism and the Theory of Mind (Learning Development and Change)*. Cambridge, MA: MIT Press.

11 Article at http://hanen.org by Lauren Lowry, *Are Two Languages Better Than One?*

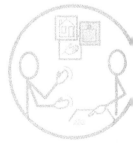

Chapter 3

The diversity of the AAC population

Before examining atypical language development in the next chapter, we will consider some of the more common developmental difficulties seen in children. We will then look at degenerative and acquired conditions in adults.

Developmental disorders

Cerebral Palsy (CP)

Cerebral Palsy[1] is a general term for a number of neurological conditions that affect movement and coordination. It is usually caused by injury to the brain before, during or after birth. There are three broad types of CP. Spastic CP is where the muscle tone is tight, causing decreased range of movement. Dyskinetic CP is where muscle movements are uncontrolled and involuntary. Ataxic CP is where the correct sequence of movements cannot be activated, resulting in unsteady, shaky movement. Most people present with mixed CP, with a combination of types. Their CP may affect four limbs, or there may be hemiplegia, with just one side of the body being affected. In some cases, just one limb is affected.

There are other associated conditions, which may or may not be present. These include learning difficulties, epilepsy, visual impairment, hearing impairment and feeding difficulties. The CP population is diverse, and it is important to build a profile of abilities for each individual person.

Because of the diversity within the CP population, communication and language development is very individual. Many people with CP are cognitively able, and despite their very different physical and sensory experiences of the world, they develop receptive language relatively easily.

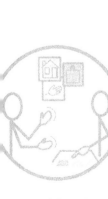

Some people with mild CP develop good functional speech. Others need AAC as their main means of expressive language. Some people with CP have learning disabilities or language-processing difficulties, and so need AAC to support receptive language too. Because it is unclear in the first few years how severely an individual is affected, it is best practice to introduce AAC early. This is likely to be symbol-based initially, with a view to becoming text-based as literacy develops.

Because of motor impairments, direct access though finger-pointing or fist-pointing may not be the best access method, and so indirect access via one or two switches should be explored early. An Occupational Therapist should be consulted to help find the most suitable switch access method. Eye-gaze technology may be an option, but switch skills are always worth developing concurrently, as eye-gaze is an extremely tiring access method, and you have to be very good at it to use it for communication.[2]

Down Syndrome

Down Syndrome[3] is a genetic condition resulting from trisomy of chromosome 21, resulting in learning disability. Individuals are also likely to have reduced muscle tone, heart defects and conductive hearing loss.

There is great diversity within the Down Syndrome population, so that some individuals develop intelligible speech, while some will need sign and symbol support throughout their lives. Children will tend to follow the same order of language acquisition, but there will be a delay. Higher language functions such as reasoning and abstract language may not be achieved. In common with many children with learning difficulties, children with Down Syndrome tend to be visual learners, and respond well to the early introduction of signs and symbols, to support attention and listening skills, and receptive as well as expressive language. People with Down Syndrome tend to have good literacy outcomes with the right intervention.

Autism Spectrum Condition (ASC)

Also known as Autism Spectrum Disorder (ASD),[4] and including high-functioning autism, or Asperger's Syndrome, this is a developmental condition which affects how people experience the world and interact with others. The sensory experiences of people with ASC are different, in that some sensory stimuli are overwhelming, and others barely perceived. This can vary from day to day and hour to hour. People with autism struggle to relate to other people,[5] and this can affect their non-verbal communication and the development of spoken language. There is wide variation within these domains. Some children do not develop spoken language and have limited intentional communication. Some children have advanced spoken language, but struggle with the social rules of communication and non-literal language. Children with ASC benefit from visual support, which provides structure in a confusing sensory and social world.

Global Delay and Learning Difficulties

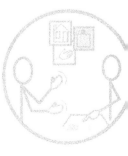

A child who does not reach a number of early developmental milestones on time (e.g. smiling, sitting, crawling, walking, talking) may be described as "globally delayed".[6] The reason may not be understood, or the child may be diagnosed with a specific genetic condition or syndrome. After the age of 5, Global Delay tends to be referred to as "Learning Disability". Cognitive tests may classify the learning disability as "mild", "moderate" or "severe", or there may be Profound Multiple Learning Disability (PMLD), including sensory and motor impairments. Individuals with learning difficulties will need more support to acquire new skills. A child with mild or moderate learning difficulties may follow the same order of language acquisition, but progress more slowly. A child with severe or profound multiple disability will experience more disruption in the acquisition of skills. There is enormous diversity within this population, but all will benefit from early introduction of sign and symbol support alongside spoken and written language.

Sensory Impairment (Visual, Hearing or Multiple)[7]

It is unusual for a child to be completely blind or deaf. Children are likely to be able to make use of what vision or hearing they have, and this can be optimised with glasses, hearing aids or cochlear implants. Sensory Impairment may be associated with other neurological conditions such as Cerebral Palsy or genetic disorders. If there is one sensory impairment with no other disability, the child is likely to acquire language normally. This will be spoken language in the case of visual impairment, and British Sign Language (BSL) in the case of profound hearing impairment. Language acquisition is likely to be more affected if there is an additional impairment, be it sensory, motor, cognitive or social communication.

During the first year or two of life, the child's level of sensory impairment may not be known. We should assume that they will be able to make use of some sensory information from each of these channels. In the case of visual impairment, reciprocity (the ability to mirror the facial expressions and body language of others) and joint-attention (the ability to share a focus of interest with another person) are likely to be affected, but these skills can be learnt through tactile and auditory communication. Parents of visually impaired children tend to intuitively take objects to the baby's body, so that the baby can feel and hear them. Similarly, a hearing impaired child may be able to "feel" their parents' voice on their body, and noise-makers may vibrate so that the child can feel them and use what hearing they have. Hearing impaired children will tend to make more use of visual information, and signing should be introduced early. We should make observations, based on caregivers' reports, about what sort of sensory stimulation the child tends to respond to or prefer. Dynamic assessment[8] can help fine-tune AAC access methods.

Developmental Verbal Dyspraxia (DVD)

Children with Developmental Verbal Dyspraxia have difficulty making the precise motor movements for speech. They have difficulty producing individual sounds, and sequencing those sounds to make words and phrases. There may also be generalised dyspraxia, affecting gross and fine motor patterns in the rest of the body. Children with DVD have unimpaired receptive language, and are able to compose correct sentences, but do not have the physical coordination to say them. Children with DVD may be helped by sign and symbol support to augment their spoken and written language.

Specific Language Impairment (SLI)

Specific Language Impairment[9] affects the development of receptive and expressive language skills, which may include learning new words, or understanding or producing complex sentences. Children with SLI have normal non-verbal cognitive abilities. This population requires early intensive intervention, and children typically benefit from early introduction of signs and symbols to support spoken and written language. Like DVD, the SLI population is relatively new to the AAC world, but in our clinical experience, responds extremely well to high-tech symbol- and text-based support, as children can see how vocabulary is organised, how phrases and sentences are constructed, and how phonemes are combined to make words.

Acquired and degenerative conditions

So far we have talked about developmental disorders that may lead to a need for AAC. We will now look at acquired and degenerative conditions.

There is an important clinical distinction between AAC users who have a developmental condition and those who have an acquired or degenerative condition. The first group are acquiring language atypically, but will make progress. The second group acquired language in a typical way, and have been competent spoken language users. This will usually support their AAC use. Some individuals with acquired conditions will remain stable, while some will improve and even recover. Individuals with degenerative conditions vary in the rate and pattern of deterioration. The AAC solution therefore will need to be responsive to changing needs. There may be more resistance to AAC, because it is a slower and more effortful communication method, and the individual is used to spoken language being instantaneous and automatic. This needs acknowledgement and sensitive handling.

Head and brain injury[10]

This might be as a result of a head injury, a stroke or a tumour. Symptoms vary depending on the part of the brain affected. There may be temporary or permanent cognitive, physical, sensory or language impairments. Aphasia is the term for this

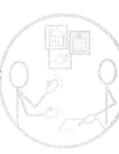

type of acquired language impairment, which may affect any part of receptive or expressive spoken or written language. These difficulties may be quite discrete (e.g. the person can write a word but cannot say it). Therefore highly individualised AAC solutions are needed.

Head and neck cancer[11]

This may include temporary loss of voice as a result of radiotherapy, or could be permanent loss of voice in the case of laryngectomy. An electrolarynx or speaking valve may be suitable, allowing the patient to continue to use their own speech. If this is not possible, then a text-to-speech communication app may be used. The individual will have unimpaired cognition and language skills.

Degenerative conditions in childhood

Rett Syndrome

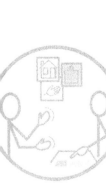

Rett Syndrome[12] is a rare condition predominantly affecting girls. Signs typically appear in the first 6–12 months, including Global Delay, low muscle tone, feeding difficulties and abnormal hand movements. There is then a rapid regression between 1 and 4 years. Repetitive hand movements take over, there are periods of severe distress, social withdrawal, and sleep and eating difficulties. There is often a plateau between 2 and 10 years, with some symptoms improving. This stage can last for many years. Scoliosis in the spine and spasticity in the legs may occur in the final stage.

Muscular Dystrophy

Muscular Dystrophy[13] is a group of muscle-wasting conditions, including Duchenne Muscular Dystrophy. These conditions vary in severity, with Duchenne being severe, but even within this condition there is considerable variation. In Duchenne Muscular Dystrophy, legs will weaken between 7 and 11 years, and the child may lose the ability to walk. Between 12 and 14, arms may become weaker. Heart and breathing problems and scoliosis occur from 16 years, and these may be treated with steroids or surgery. A ventilator may be needed in the person's twenties or thirties.

Degenerative conditions in adulthood

Motor Neurone Disease

Motor Neurone Disease (MND)[14] describes a group of progressive neurodegenerative diseases which attack the motor neurones and lead to weakness and wasting of muscles. Those muscles first affected tend to be in the hands, feet and mouth. There is later loss of mobility as limbs are affected, and there are difficulties with speech, swallowing and breathing. Senses are not generally affected. Some people experience cognitive and behaviour change. MND tends to progress very rapidly, and so referral to Specialised AAC Assessment Hub Centres[15] should be immediate, and will be prioritised.

Multiple Sclerosis

Multiple Sclerosis (MS)[16] is a group of conditions of the central nervous system. The specific symptoms that appear depend upon which part of the nervous system is affected, but can include problems with balance, vision, fatigue, bladder and bowel, stiffness of movement, tremor, swallowing, speech, memory or cognition. The progression of MS varies, and can be relapsing-remitting or progressive.

Parkinson's Disease

Parkinson's Disease[17] is a progressive neurological condition whereby there is a reduction of dopamine in the brain, leading to tremor, slow movements and stiff and inflexible muscles. There can also be tiredness, depression, balance and memory problems. Speech and communication are affected later. Progression rates vary considerably. Parkinson's Plus Syndromes include Multiple Systems Atrophy (MSA) and Progressive Supranuclear Palsy (PSP).

Alzheimer's Disease

Alzheimer's Disease[18] is the most common cause of dementia. The chemistry and structure of the brain changes, causing memory loss and difficulties with thinking, problem-solving and language. Mood change, anxiety and depression are common. Alzheimer's is progressive. Most people get Alzheimer's over the age of 65, but there are cases of early-onset dementia. This population tends to be under-represented in AAC intervention, as interventions to support memory are often prioritised.[19]

Huntingdon's Disease

Huntingdon's Disease[20] is a hereditary neurological disease which affects movement, cognition, behaviour and language. The behaviour and social communication aspect is likely to be helped by AAC.

A summary of the AAC population

According to Communication Matters[21] and the Royal College of Speech and Language Therapy,[22] 97.5% of the total number of people who could benefit from AAC have nine conditions. These are shown in the pie chart in Figure 3.1.

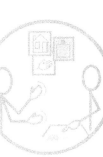

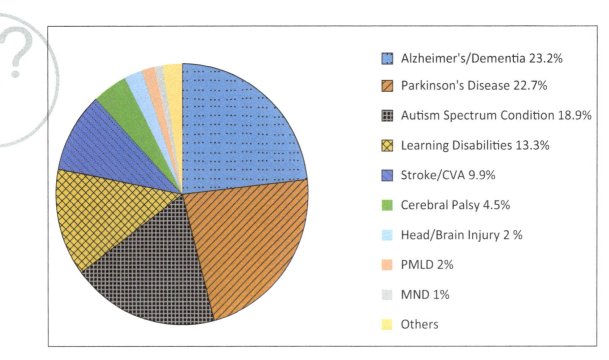

Figure 3.1 AAC users and their conditions

Coming to terms with diagnosis

Grief is significant when a child has a developmental disorder. Some conditions can be diagnosed in utero or at birth (e.g. Down Syndrome). Other conditions, like Cerebral Palsy, may be suspected if there has been premature or difficult birth, and these babies will be closely monitored. Diagnosis may not be made until the end of the first year or into the second year. Conditions such as Autism Spectrum Condition and Global Developmental Delay may not be diagnosed until later.

Parents often report falling into a "black hole" following diagnosis as they try to absorb life-changing news. It is a time when they receive a lot of information, but may be unable to process it all. This is a good time to signpost families to organisations which support those with the same conditions.

Parents of children with developmental difficulties report going through stages in grief, with some key life stages being particularly painful. However there will be great variation in parents' reactions to diagnoses, and professionals must be sensitive and respectful of parents' emotions.

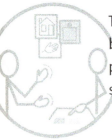

The families of children with significant developmental conditions will typically be offered Early Support.[23] Early Support offers a network of professional support, practical resources, training and a key-worker to coordinate health and therapy services.

The diagnosis of an acquired or degenerative condition will be a terrible shock to the affected individual and their family. There may be significant adjustments to be made in work and lifestyle, with impacts on self-image and relationships. It is vital that those affected are signposted to sources of support, including local groups and national associations for their particular condition.

The emotional impact of a diagnosis may affect management of AAC. Generally, parents of children with developmental conditions have concerns over whether AAC will prevent their child from speaking. Those with degenerative conditions may not want to consider a time in the future when they will not be able to speak. These issues will need very sensitive handling. It is important that families receive accurate information based on research and best practice guidelines so that they can make an informed decision.

Child and adult safeguarding

In (rare) cases where there is disagreement about the best treatment for an individual, Child or Adult Safeguarding[24] procedures may need to be implemented. Always seek advice from relevant Safeguarding Professionals in your organisation to ensure that you follow Local and National Guidelines. Mental Capacity[25] will need to be considered for young people and adults.

AAC for advocacy

Speech and Language Therapists and AAC professionals have a significant role to play in advocacy for children and vulnerable adults. They are best placed to advise other services how the individual communicates and which strategies to use to allow their voice to be heard. Communication Passports[26] and opinion charts such as *Talking Mats*[27] (see Chapter 5 for more details) may be used for advocacy.

Notes

1 See http://scope.org.uk for more information.
2 See Chapter 7 for more information about switches and eye-gaze for access.
3 See http://downs-syndrome.org.uk for more information.
4 See http://autism.org.uk for more information.
5 See Baron-Cohen, S. (1995) *Mindblindness: An Essay in Autism and Theory of Mind*. Cambridge, MA: MIT Press.
6 See http://mencap.org.uk for more information.
7 See http://sense.org.uk for more information.
8 See Chapter 10 for more information on dynamic assessment.
9 See http://ican.org.uk for more information.
10 See http://headway.org.uk for more information.
11 See http://macmillan.org.uk for more information.

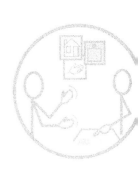

12 See http://rettuk.org for more information.

13 See http://musculardystrophyuk.org for more information.

14 See http://mndassociation.org for more information.

15 See Chapter 10 for more information about AAC Hubs.

16 See http://mssociety.org.uk for more information.

17 See http://parkinsons.org.uk for more information.

18 See http://alzheimers.org.uk for more information.

19 Beukelman, D., Fager, S., Ball, L. and Dietz, A. (2007) AAC for adults with acquired neurological conditions: A review. *Augmentative and Alternative Communication*, 23(3), 230–242.

20 See http://has.org.uk for more information.

21 Communication Matters (2013) *Shining a Light on Augmentative and Alternative Communication*. Communication Matters Research Matters: An AAC Evidence Base Research Project – Final Report, on http://communicationmatters.org.uk website.

22 http://rcslt.org. *Augmentative and Alternative Communication: Prevalence and Incidence*, online resource for members of the RCLST.

23 See the National Children's Bureau website, http://ncb.org.uk, for more information about *Early Support*.

24 See www.gov.uk for *Safeguarding Children and Young People* and *Safeguarding Policy: Protecting Vulnerable Adults*, policy papers, which have links to relevant guidance in the UK.

25 See www.gov.uk for *Mental Capacity Act 2005 Code of Practice* (2007) for information on Lasting Power of Attorney (LPA), Court of Protection and Mental Capacity Advocates.

26 http://communicationpassports.org.uk.

27 http://talkingmats.com.

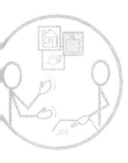

Chapter 4

Atypical language development and acquired disorders

In Chapter 2 we looked at Typical Language Development. We will now consider Atypical Language Development.

There has been extensive research into the acquisition of spoken language in typically developing children.[1] Practitioners generally agree on developmental norms, which were outlined in the previous section.

There has been some research into the acquisition of spoken language in children with delayed and disordered language.[2] Delayed language means that the child goes through the same stages of language development (e.g. first words emerge before two-word combinations), but the process is slower. In disordered language, there may be a mismatch between skill areas. For example, vocabulary acquisition may be less impaired than grammar, or vice versa.

There is less research into the acquisition of language where augmentative and alternative communication is used. Some studies have tracked the development of Makaton signs in children who have learning difficulties.[3] Early studies into symbol use tended to focus on a small group of individuals over a very short period.[4] More recently there have been studies which track small groups of individuals over a longer time-frame.[5] These studies are beginning to show the different rate or order of acquisition of various aspects of language, including vocabulary, grammar and social use of language.

For detailed reviews and discussion around research to date, see Light, Beukelman and Reichle[6] and Von Tetzchner and Grove.[7]

We have seen already the diversity of the AAC population. Von Tetzchner and Martinsen[8] describe three broad categories of AAC users:

1   Expressive Language Group: individuals with relatively unimpaired cognition and receptive language, but who have neuromotor impairment affecting body movements and/or speech (e.g. Cerebral Palsy with no learning difficulty).

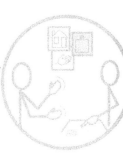

2 Supportive Group: individuals requiring temporary AAC support (e.g. transient language delay), or those who only need AAC in certain communicative situations (e.g. Autism Spectrum Condition).

3 Alternative Language Group: individuals who need AAC support for both receptive and expressive language development (e.g. Learning Difficulties).

These three groups are likely to follow different trajectories in their acquisition of spoken language and AAC communication. In the future, AAC support may be tailored to the differing needs of these groups, and they may follow distinct care pathways. For example, those in the expressive language group may need less formal language teaching, but more support with access to AAC. Those in the alternative language group may need more visual support for their receptive language acquisition as well as for their expressive language.

With more research, distinct patterns of acquisition may emerge, depending on factors including the child's overall diagnosis, their individual patterns of physical, sensory, cognitive, language or social communication abilities or impairments, the quality of the communication or language input, and the AAC solutions selected for them. Following are some of the differences a child may experience in atypical language acquisition.

The child's sensory-motor experience of the world

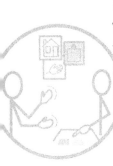

A child with Visual Impairment or Hearing Impairment will experience the world very differently from a child who does not. Different neuronal connections will be made, and different patterns of experience and analysis will take place. Similarly, a child with difficulties moving around and manipulating objects will develop concepts differently. How things look, sound, feel, taste and smell; how this changes when viewed from different perspectives; how objects move and what we can do with them, all contribute to our semantic knowledge. The varied numbers of ways that referrants can interact with one another contribute to our syntactic knowledge, for example "ball in the box", "ball out of the box", "roll the ball", "kick the ball", "kick the ball into the box", "the ball rolled out of the box".

It seems reasonable to assume that anything that affects our experience of the world will affect our semantic and syntactic development. Therefore there is a need for early intervention to allow children with sensory and motor impairment to access and explore the physical environment.[9] Using switch-operated toys may help these children to develop cause-and-effect and reduce later passivity.[10]

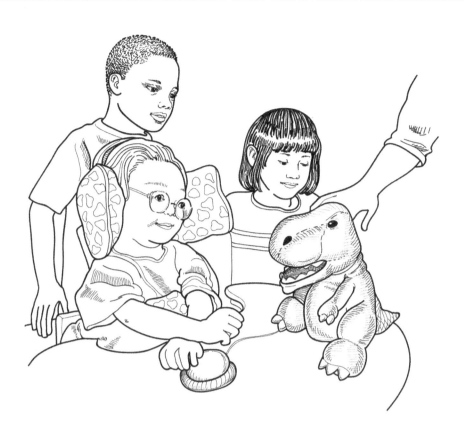

Joint-attention and AAC

In typical language development, when a child is learning to attend to a word, they have to shift their attention from the object they are interested in, to the word that the caregiver says. In AAC language development, the child has to shift their attention from the object they are interested in, to the word that the caregiver says, to the symbol they are pointing at (or sign they are producing). This is an extra demand on their attention.[11] We can help by making it as easy as possible for the child to see us and the symbol or sign. Typically developing children soon learn to integrate looking and listening so that they no longer have to shift their gaze to the adult to register the spoken word. We need to position our AAC input so that the child does not have to perform conscious gaze-shifts. Eventually we hope that their gaze-shift will become automatic.

Spoken language input

It is unclear from the research literature how the quality or quantity of language input differs for children with developmental delays. There is some evidence to suggest that there is reduced language input, because more time is spent on care-giving activities than on play and interaction,[12] or different types of input, with directives being more frequent (possibly because of increased care routines),[13] and with more language around social play and less around object play.[14] Researchers

disagree about whether the reduced input is helpful or not. The optimal amount of spoken input is probably different for different children. Interventions such as *Parent-Child Interaction*[15] may be helpful in establishing what is right for an individual child.

AAC modelling

In typical language acquisition, children are exposed to modelling from competent spoken language users. In AAC acquisition, children are exposed to modelling from adults who are also just learning the AAC language themselves. The research suggests that early intervention should focus on parents, so that they provide a rich language input throughout all communication contexts.[16] *Aided Language Stimulation*[17] is where caregivers model AAC as part of this language input. This will be discussed in more detail in Chapter 9.

Vocabulary size, combining symbols and communicative functions

By the time a typically developing child is 3 years old, they typically have an expressive vocabulary of 3,000 words.[18] A child using AAC will have a much smaller expressive (and possibly receptive) vocabulary size. It has been suggested that children need a critical mass of vocabulary in order to make the generalisations that are needed for grammar to develop.[19] Certainly, children seem to need at least 50 words before they can combine words. Children also need multiple opportunities to combine and re-combine words[20] to create novel utterances that convey multiple meanings. Adults will need to interpret these. There is some evidence in the research literature that adults tend to assume that AAC users are making requests when they may in fact be commenting, or telling the adult about something that has happened or going to happen.[21] The child who uses AAC is more reliant on an adult interpreting their utterance, doing so in an attuned way, and being sensitive to the variety of communicative functions the child may want to convey.

Making use of typical language acquisition

In the absence of detailed research data, it seems fair for now to rely on clinical observations. This suggests that children acquiring non-spoken language tend to go through the same broad sequence of language acquisition.

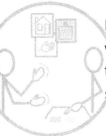

For example, in terms of vocabulary, we tend to assume that nouns come before verbs. In terms of syntax, we assume that that single signs or symbols come before two-sign or two-symbol combinations. In terms of social use of language, we tend to see that requesting comes before commenting.

We can therefore set targets for children based on the typical order of acquisition of language, provided we are giving children the appropriate tools and the varied opportunities to achieve these targets. If we want a child to combine symbols, we need to give them a wide vocabulary, and this vocabulary needs to reflect the child's activities and interests. We need to model multiple examples of how to combine these symbols and offer opportunities for the child to play and experiment with combining symbols.

We must acknowledge that this is a working-model of atypical language development, and that there may be considerable variation within the AAC population, given that they are a diverse group with a wide range of sensory, motor, cognitive and social communication experiences.

Gathering more evidence

Perhaps the way forward is a lot more single-case studies or small group studies, examining factors including the various modes of communication available to these individuals, the quantity and quality of modelling or teaching, and their various abilities or impairments. Long-term studies, which track progress over many years, might be particularly helpful.

Communication Matters, the UK charity for AAC, now has an AAC Evidence Base website.[22] This includes theory-driven publications and practice-driven interventions, including single case studies. A case study template and database provides information for researchers. Communication Matters continues to collaborate with AAC users, universities and stakeholders to promote research and the sharing of best practices.

An immediate measure that clinicians can use in managing an individual case is to keep detailed records of a child's current multi-modal communication. Sampling this at regular intervals provides some evidence of how language is progressing in various domains. See the *AAC Transcription Record* in Chapter 11 for an example of how to record current AAC use.

A receptive-expressive gap

In typical spoken language development, there is a seamless transition between non-verbal communication in the first year of life and access to spoken communication from the second year of life. The nature of many developmental difficulties, with the exception of Down Syndrome, and perhaps Cerebral Palsy, is that a diagnosis of developmental difficulties may not be made until the second or third year, or later. The child's access to an alternative means of expression, that is signs and symbols, may therefore be delayed.

We know that there are "windows of development" in language acquisition. In rare cases where unimpaired children have had no access to spoken language, we know that even if spoken language is introduced at a later age, the child is unlikely to achieve mastery of it. What if we miss this window of development in aided language development? The same child could have made a smooth transition into aided expressive language, but instead is held back while there is uncertainty about whether they will develop spoken language.

I would never say to a parent that their child will not develop spoken language. This takes away all hope. There have been many children who I have worked with, particularly within the ASC population, who have not shown any signs of developing spoken language, with no signs of babble, at 5 years old. However, by 8 years old they have fluent spoken language. We therefore can never say never. BUT, while we continue to model spoken language, the earlier we introduce an alternative means of expressive language, the better. In this way, we do not risk the child being caught in limbo when they are ready to start experimenting with expression but have no means to do so.

When to introduce AAC

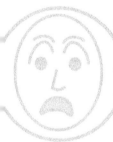

Where there is a possibility that an infant will have a developmental delay, for example in the case of a known condition or where the infant is premature, the best practice is to encourage the caregiver to become attuned to the infant's communicative signals as early as possible. The caregiver should be provided with information about language acquisition and the prerequisites for communication, just as they are provided with information about feeding, sleeping and positioning. Many Special Care Baby Units (SCBU) have outreach services once babies are discharged from the hospital, with specialist nurses providing home visits to continue to support caregivers in caring for these infants.

Studies have shown that caregivers can recognise and encourage infants' pre-intentional communicative signals as early as 8 months.[23] In a research review, Branson and Demchak[24] concluded that

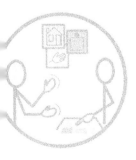

a variety of AAC methods can be effective when caregivers respond contingently and consistently to the child's communicative attempts. If a toddler's natural gestures are difficult to interpret, a clinician should not hesitate to introduce pictures or a VOCA (Voice Output Communication Aid)[25] in order to increase the caregiver's ability to recognise and respond to the child's communicative attempts. Furthermore the clinician should be willing to try a variety of AAC methods.

As early as possible, at six months ideally, we could be exposing this child to signs and symbols. It has become more common to use "baby signs" with the typically developing population. Research suggests that babies benefit from this type of input, with caregivers becoming more attuned to their babies' non-verbal communication.[26] There may be short-term and long-term gains in receptive and expressive language.[27]

Alongside spoken language, we can sign key words with a baby. We can show single symbols in the same way. We might start to label the child's home with a few symbols: drawers and cupboards might be labelled with "T-shirt", "trousers", "cup", "spoon". We might match a symbol to a photo of "mummy" and "daddy", or pictures in a book of "dog" and "cat". We might have a little key-ring of core words in symbol format (e.g. "more", "gone", "help", "no").

We might introduce choices of two or more symbols. We might introduce simple communication charts to go with specific activities, such as bath time, playing with bubbles, a ball, bricks, playdough or a doll. We might have communication charts for choosing a song or sharing a book (see Chapter 5 for examples of these). We might have physical ways of combining individual symbols, for example attaching them to a sentence strip, if it is felt that pointing to symbols in turn is not enough.

Light and Drager[28] have carried out research into introducing VOCAs for very young children. They explored the use of *Visual Scene Displays*. Visual Scene Displays consist of photos of the child and their family carrying out interesting activities, with areas called "hotspots" on the screen, which, when activated, speak relevant social phrases and words. When these were used in fun, interactive games, there were significant early communication gains. These included increased participation in communicative exchanges, increased turns, and the ability to progress to other types of AAC display, including traditional grid layouts of symbols or text. There are now some very exciting vocabulary packages for very young children which utilize Visual Scene Displays. The child can then move on to hybrid packages which utilize both Visual Scene Displays and traditional symbol- or text-based grids. These are explored in Chapter 6.

Text-based communication using spelling offers infinite scope for creative conversation. We need to plan for literacy development from early on. The opportunity to play with speech sounds, for example by using Voice Output Communication Devices (VOCAs) offers an alternative to babbling. Adults might then scaffold words that begin the same sound. Literacy teaching will be examined in more detail in Chapter 12.

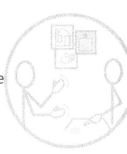

Better late than never

If a child is 3 or 5, or older, it is better to introduce AAC late than never. AAC practitioners have all come across older children or even adults who, exposed to AAC relatively late, have been able to convey complex messages using their new AAC system. It is incredibly moving to consider that these individuals had that ability locked inside them all along, but needed a means to express themselves.

Bilingualism and multilingualism and AAC

If a child's home language is not the dominant language, then it is best practice to duplicate AAC resources in both languages. Which resource to be used will be determined by which language the communication partner is proficient in, to ensure the child hears a good spoken language model in each language. For example, if a grandmother only speaks Gujarati, she will only use the Gujarati translation of the communication book. If the father only speaks English, he will use the English version. The mother may be proficient in both, but I would tend to advise she uses her first language, at least in the home.

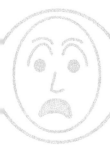

For low- and light-tech AAC, it is advised that the child's family help to translate the written text accompanying symbols. Resources such as *Google Translate* can be very approximate in their translations, and so this method is not recommended. Some high-tech vocabulary packages have been translated into many different languages. It is worth asking families to check the quality of the translation. For languages where there are many dialectal variations, it is important to choose the correct one.

Where it is known that a child has a significant Global Delay, there may be discussion about concentrating on one language. Families should not be pressured by professionals into restricting a child to English if the family does not speak English at home. However if the parents are proficient in more than one language, and English is one of these, and the child will attend an English-speaking school, there is a stronger argument for concentrating on English. The Speech and Language Therapist should provide the family with information about bilingual and multilingual language development so that they can make an informed decision. A second language may be introduced later, or key words or phrases may still be taught.

Notes

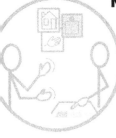

1 Bloom, L. (1993) *The Transition From Infancy to Language: Acquiring the Power of Expression.* Cambridge, UK: Cambridge University Press; Bloom, L. (2000) *How Children Learn the Meanings of Words.* Cambridge, MA: MIT Press; Bruner, J. (1983) *Child's Talk: Learning to Use Language.* Oxford, UK: Oxford University Press.

2 Bishop, D.V.M. (1997) *Uncommon Understanding: Development and Disorders of Language Understanding in Children*. Hove, UK: Psychology Press.

3 For example, Grove, N. and Dockerell, J. (2000) Multi-sign combinations by children with intellectual impairments: An analysis of language skills. *Journal of Language, Speech and Hearing Research*, 43, 309–323.

4 Light, J. (1985) *The Communicative Interaction Patterns of Non-Speaking Physically Disabled Children and their Primary Caregivers*. Toronto, Canada: Blissymbolics Communication Institute; Von Tetzchner, S. and Martinsen, H. (1996) Words and Strategies: Conversations with young children who use aided language. In S. Von Tetzchner and H. Martinsen (eds.) (2000) *Augmentative and Alternative Communication: European Perspectives*. London: Whurr, pp. 65–88.

5 Lund, S. and Light, J. (2001) *Fifteen Years Later: An Investigation of the Long-Term Outcomes of Augmentative and Alternative Communication Interventions* (Student-Initiated Research Grant HB24B990069). University Park: Pennsylvania State University.

6 Light, J., Beukelman, D. and Reichle, J. (2003) *Communicative Competence for Individuals Who Use AAC: From Research to Effective Practice*. Baltimore: Paul H. Brookes.

7 Von Tetzchner and Grove (eds.) (2003) *Augmentative and Alternative Communication: Developmental Disorders*. London: Whurr.

8 Von Tetzchner, S. and Martinsen, H. (2000) *Augmentative and Alternative Communication*. London: Whurr.

9 Blockberger, S. and Sutton, A. (2003) Language experiences and knowledge of children with extremely limited speech. In Light, J., Beukelman, D. and Reichle, J. (eds.), *Communicative Competence for Individuals Who Use AAC: From Research to Effective Practice*. Baltimore: Paul H. Brookes, p. 95.

10 Iacono, T. (2003) Pragmatic development in individuals with developmental disabilities who use AAC. In Light, J., Beukelman, D. and Reichle, J. (eds.), *Communicative Competence for Individuals Who Use AAC: From Research to Effective Practice*. Baltimore: Paul H. Brookes, p. 345.

11 Hunt-Beg, M. (1998) *Children's Use of Pointing Cues in Aided Language Intervention*. Paper presented at the Eighth Biennial Conference of the International Society for Augmentative and Alternative Communication (ISAAC), Dublin, Ireland.

12 Calculator, S. (1997) Fostering early language acquisition and AAC use: Exploring reciprocal influences between children and their environments. *Augmentative and Alternative Communication*, 3, 149–157.

13 Light, J. and Kelford Smith, A. (1993) Home literacy experiences of pre-schoolers who use AAC systems and of their non-disabled peers. *Augmentative and Alternative Communication*, 9, 10–25.

14 Cress, C., Linke, M., Moskall, L., Benal, A., Anderson, V. and LaMontagne, J. (2000, November) *Play and Parent Interaction in Young Children with Physical Impairments*. Paper presented at the conference of American Speech-Language-Hearing Association, Washington, DC.

15 See Chapter 9 for a brief discussion of parent-based interventions and Aided Language Stimulation.

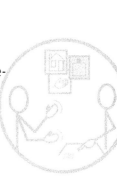

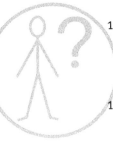

16 Blockberger, S. and Sutton, A. (2003) Language experiences and knowledge of children with extremely limited speech. In Light, J., Beukelman, D. and Reichle, J. (eds.), *Communicative Competence for Individuals Who Use AAC: From Research to Effective Practice*. Baltimore: Paul H. Brookes, p. 95.

17 Romski, M. and Sevcik, R. (2003) Enhancing communication development. In Light, J., Beukelman, D. and Reichle, J. (eds.), *Communicative Competence for Individuals Who Use AAC: From Research to Effective Practice*. Baltimore: Paul H. Brookes.

18 Mehrabian, A. (1970) Measures of vocabulary and grammatical skills for children up to age 6. *Developmental Psychology*, 2(3), 439–446.

19 Sutton, A. (1999) Language learning experiences and grammatical acquisition. In Loncke, F., Clibbens, J., Arvidson, H. and Lloyd, L. (eds.), *Augmentative and Alternative Communication: New Directions in Research and Practice*. San Diego: Whurr.

20 Nelson, N. (1992) Performance is the prize: Language competence and performance among AAC users. *Augmentative and Alternative Communication*, 8, 3–18.

21 Blockberger, S. and Sutton, A. (2003) Language experiences and knowledge of children with extremely limited speech. In Light, J., Beukelman, D. and Reichle, J. (eds.), *Communicative Competence for Individuals Who Use AAC: From Research to Effective Practice*. Baltimore: Paul H. Brookes.

22 http://aacknowledge.org.uk.

23 Chen, D., Klein, D. and Haney, M. (2007) Promoting Interactions with infants who have complex multiple disabilities: field-testing of the PLAI curriculum. *Infants and Young Children: An Interdisciplinary Journal of Special Care Practices*, 20, 149–162.

24 Branson, D. and Demchak, M. (2009) The use of augmentative and alternative communication methods with infants and toddlers with disabilities: A research review. *Augmentative and Alternative Communication*, 25(4), 274–286.

25 In the United States, Voice Output Communication Aids (VOCAs) are referred to as Speech Generating Devices (SGDs).

26 Johnston, J., Durieux-Smith, A. and Bloom, K. (2005) Teaching gestural signs to infants to advance child development. *First Language*, 25, 235–251.

27 Goodwyn, S., Acredolo, L. and Brown, C. A. (2000) Impact of symbolic gesturing on early language development. *Journal of Nonverbal Behavior*, 24, 81–103.

28 Light, J. and Drager, K. (2007) AAC technologies for young children with complex communication needs: State of the science and future research directions. *Augmentative and Alternative Communication*, 23, 204–216.

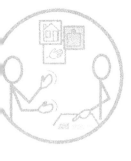

Chapter 5

No-tech, low-tech and light-tech AAC

In the next two chapters, I will explain four types of AAC: no-tech, low-tech, light-tech and high-tech. Before I do that, I will examine photographs and symbol sets. In Chapter 10 we will consider how you choose an AAC solution for an individual client. For all of these solutions, make use of the professionals working with the child. If a child has a visual impairment, then work with their VI Specialist Teacher. If a child has a hearing impairment, then work with their HI Specialist Teacher and Speech and Language Therapist. If the child has a physical impairment, then work with their Physiotherapist and Occupational Therapist.

Photographs

These initially seem like a good place to start. A potential AAC user may show more interest in photographs than in symbols. There is some evidence to suggest that very young AAC users engage more with high-tech AAC if Visual Scene Displays are used. These include photographs of the AAC user themselves and their family.[1] However, for many of the low-tech solutions explored in this section, photographs have to be very clear, with the main focus of the photograph (e.g. a cup) clearly visible against a plain white background. Problems may arise if the cup in the photo is different to the real cup being used. From the start, a symbol is more abstract, and stands for any number of cups. If a potential AAC user can manage this level of abstraction, and most can, then symbols are a better solution than photographs. Photographs have their place, for example for specific people and toys, but it is time-consuming to make a communication chart or book made only of photographs.

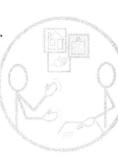

Some AAC users become very distracted by photographs of people in their AAC system. There is an argument for using symbols for important people rather than photographs. However, this will need to be decided with the individual and their family.

Consent for photographs of people must always be sought. Consider the data protection implications when transferring and storing photographs electronically. Photos should only be emailed to and from secure addresses; encryption should be used with laptops and memory sticks; files should be securely stored in one location and deleted from devices when not needed.

Symbol sets

There are three symbol sets that are widely used in the UK and that are included in symbol software and AAC resources. These are Widgit Literacy Symbols (WLS), Picture Communication Symbols (PCS) and SymbolStix. I will consider these first, and then I will consider some other symbol sets that are also in use, but with specific resources.

Widgit Literacy Symbols (WLS)

These can be colour or black-and-white. There are 15,000 symbols available. This is a UK symbol set, originally called Rebus, and developed by Widgit. Additional visually impaired symbols are available for the visually impaired population. These are used in symbol resource-making software including *SymWriter* and *InPrint 3*, in curriculum software including *Clicker 7*, and in all of the *Grid 3* vocabulary packages. WLS have tended to dominate in educational settings. There is an argument for starting children off with a symbol set that they are likely to be exposed to in their education. Skin tones can be changed. Most symbols with people are gender-neutral.

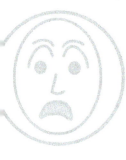

Figure 5.1 Mummy loves eating chocolate (WLS)

Widgit Symbols © Widgit Software 2002–2017 http://www.widgit.com.

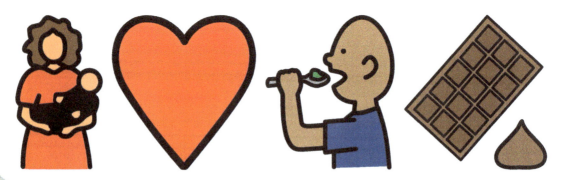

Figure 5.2 Mummy loves eating chocolate (PCS)

The Picture Communication Symbols ©1981–2017 by Tobii Dynavox. All Rights Reserved Worldwide. Used with permission. Boardmaker® is a trademark of Tobii Dynavox.

Picture Communication Symbols (PCS)

This was the first symbol set available in colour. There are over 30,000 symbols available. They were originally developed for children, and have a child-friendly, cartoony look. Additional high-contrast symbols are available for the visually impaired population, and thin-line symbols for the academic and adult markets. PCS were developed by Mayer Johnson in the US, and used in *Boardmaker*[2] symbol resource-making software. They still tend to have an American bias in the choice of vocabulary. PCS symbols tend to be more multi-function than WLS. For example, there is a symbol for "I, me, mine," where these are three separate symbols in WLS. This avoids unnecessary reduplication of vocabulary, but means that there is increased need for interpretation. Skin tone and gender can be changed to match the user.

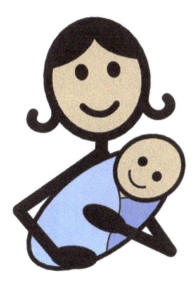

Figure 5.3 Mum (SymbolStix)

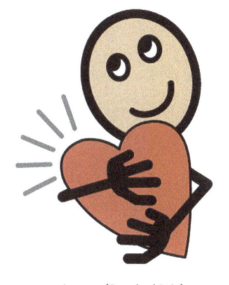

Figure 5.4 Loves (SymbolStix)

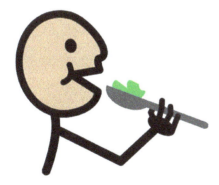

Figure 5.5 Eating (SymbolStix)

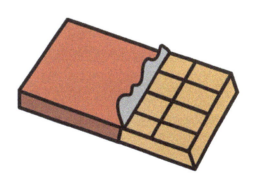

Figure 5.6 Chocolate (SymbolStix)

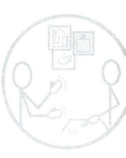

SymbolStix

There are over 30,000 colour symbols available. The symbols are described as "lively stick-people with attitude" and do have a certain charm. SymbolStix have gained popularity through the communication app *Proloquo2Go*, and are now available in symbol resource-making software including *Matrix Maker* and other vocabulary packages including *Mind Express*. Skin tones can be personalised. Actions are gender-neutral.

Makaton

Makaton have a symbol system to accompany their sign vocabulary of about 4,000 concepts. These are black-and-white only, and were designed to be easy to draw. They have language themes, such as nouns always being represented in their entirety, while verbs depict the person or part of the person carrying out the action. The ground line is used for all positional concepts, while the time line is used for all temporal concepts. While it is a beautifully designed system, Makaton has unfortunately lagged behind other symbol sets in the high-tech market. It is available as an add-in for resource-making software, but is not available for the most widely used high-tech vocabulary packages. That is not to say that it cannot catch up in the future. Makaton signs are the market leaders in the UK for manual sign resources.

Pics for PECS

PECS, the Picture Exchange Communication System,[3] is an approach used for children with Autism Spectrum Condition (ASC). PECS have produced their own symbol set of 3,200 colour pictures to accompany the programme. These include pictures of "reinforcers" that are commonly liked by learners, for example, stretchy man and spinner. The symbols are line drawings with some details. This is to reflect the literal tendencies of users, such as those who have ASC. Sentence-building is very structured, so while there are sentence starters, verbs, adjectives and prepositions alongside nouns, it might be argued that the creative use of language is limited.

Minsymbols

The Minspeak or Unity Language Programme makes use of systematic multi-meaning icons, which can be combined in different ways to make a particular word. Each combination has to be learnt by the user. The user can be taught the semantic or syntactic reasons for the choice of icons, though this is not always necessary: the pathways may be learnt by motor-planning instead.

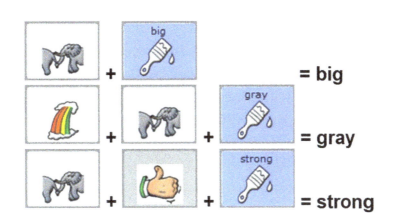

Figure 5.7 Minspeak

Bliss symbols

These are black-and-white, easy to draw, highly abstract symbols. There are over 4,500 concepts. There are language themes for type of word. Bliss symbols were once widely used with cognitively able AAC users, but fell out of favour with the emergence of PCS. Another reason they are no longer widely taught may be because there is an assumption now that cognitively able AAC users will go on to develop literacy, and so do not need an alternative highly abstract written form of language.

Making symbol resources

There are currently three main software packages for making symbol resources. These are *InPrint*[4] (WLS), *Boardmaker*[5] (PCS) and *MatrixMaker Plus*[6] (WLS and SymbolStix). They each offer templates for making communication charts and books, overlays for light-tech AAC devices, and visual supports. Additional symbol-set add-ins are available (e.g. Makaton symbols), but it is advisable to check software compatibility before purchasing.

Introducing written text

It is recommended that symbols are always accompanied by written text for children. We want to promote literacy as the ultimate aim in AAC. Symbol vocabularies are always limited, whereas the ability to spell words offers infinite possibilities of self-expression.

There is an argument that we prioritise symbols over text and should perhaps revise this practice. Always accompanying the written word with a symbol can be very distracting for beginning readers. Core words, the high-frequency words that are very abstract, like "the", "and" and "to" may be better represented by text alone. Once a child is beginning to read, it may be preferable to move them on to a hybrid text and symbol AAC system, with a view to becoming text-only. Text-only systems may make use of the alphabet for spelling, and of whole words and quick phrases.

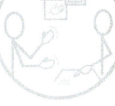

AAC users should be given access to a low-tech alphabet chart from early on. This may be in QWERTY, ABC or high-frequency layout, depending on the needs of the user. The AAC user will need frequent exposure to the alphabet and letter sounds as part of their literacy development. These should be used in conjunction with other AAC solutions, whether they are symbol-based or text-based.

Core and fringe vocabulary

In recent years, there has been much discussion in the AAC world about the use of core vocabulary.[7]

Approximately 80% of the words we speak are the 250 most frequently occurring "core" words.[8] These words occur across a range of communication contexts.[9] The words are consistent across age groups, from toddlers, to children and adults, to seniors. These words are typically the "little" words with fewer than six letters. They include pronouns (I, you), general verbs (want, get), adjectives (more, good) and adverbs (here, now). Core words dominate early language and are used in early phrase-building.

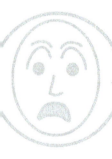

Sample core vocabulary communication charts are shown in Figures 5.8 and 5.9. The size and layout of the communication chart should reflect the individual AAC user's needs, taking into consideration the symbol set they use, their visual processing, access method, and cognitive and language abilities.

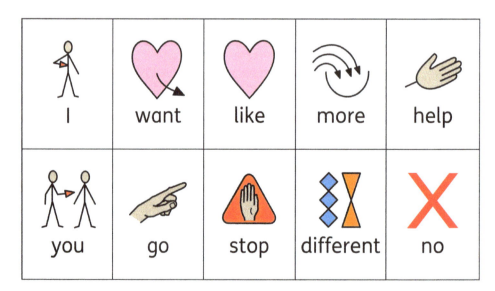

Figure 5.8 Core vocabulary communication chart (10)

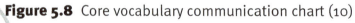

Widgit Symbols © Widgit Software 2002–2017 www.widgit.com

Core Vocabulary Communication Chart (10 cells)[10]

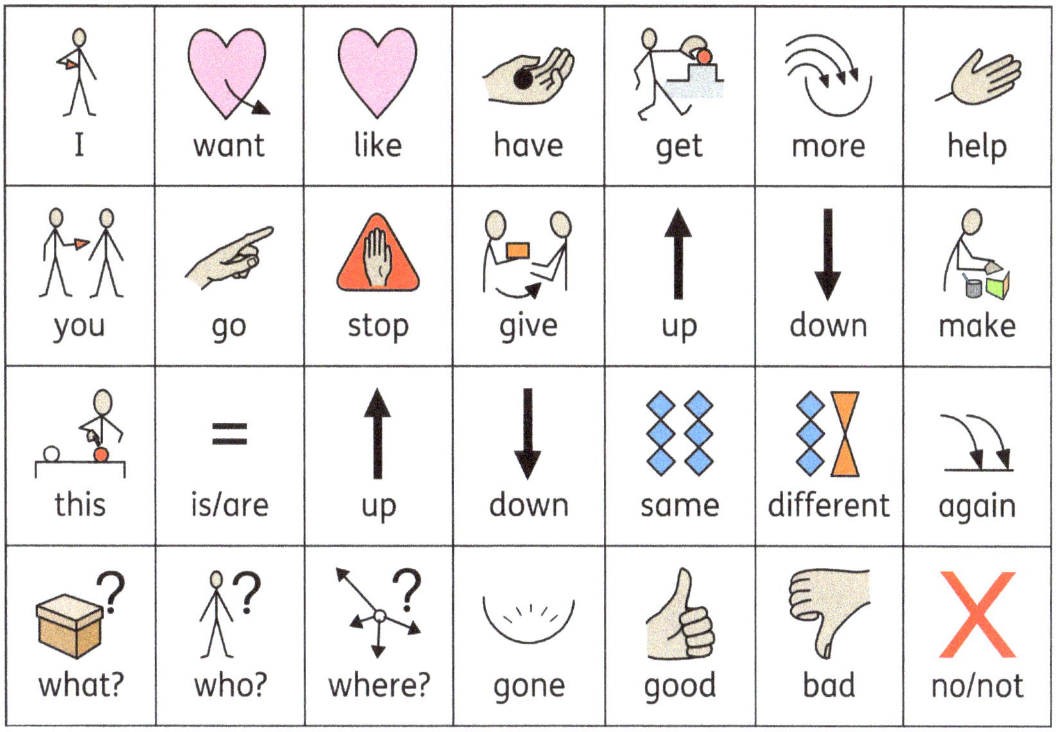

I	want	like	have	get	more	help
you	go	stop	give	up	down	make
this	is/are	up	down	same	different	again
what?	who?	where?	gone	good	bad	no/not

Figure 5.9 Core vocabulary communication chart (28)

Widgit Symbols © Widgit Software 2002–2017 www.widgit.com

Core Vocabulary Communication Chart (28 cells)[11]

It is suggested that 2–10 core words are introduced first, and more are introduced to reflect the user's pace of learning. It is helpful if those core words that have already been learnt are kept in the same positions on the page as communication charts are updated, so that the AAC user does not have to re-learn motor patterns when building phrases.

The ACE Centre[12] have a range of free downloadable communication charts on their website. This includes a range of layouts of core vocabulary and activity-based communication charts including core and fringe vocabulary. These are available for WLS, PCS and SymbolStix.

Some AAC users will be able to combine "no" or "not" with another core word, and so will not need opposite concepts. For example, instead of having "same" and "different", the user would be taught to say "not same." This saves some space on a communication chart. However this will depend on the cognitive and language level of the individual. It is very hard to generalise in AAC, as no one solution suits all users. Similarly users' needs change, so the solution evolves over time.

Core vocabulary communication charts can be used across different communication situations, so are an extremely versatile resource. It is important that all adults and settings working with an AAC user use the same grid layout, so that the AAC user does not have to re-learn locations of symbols when they move between settings.

Core words are shown in Table 5.1.[13] I have ordered these so that the most useful words in each category appear earlier in the list. However this will be personal to the user to some extent.

AAC systems can sometimes prioritise fringe words, that is, nouns. We can actually say an awful lot just with core words (try composing some messages for basic needs using those core words in Table 5.1). There is a YouTube video called *The Language*

Table 5.1 Core vocab

Pronouns	General Verbs	Specific Verbs	Adjectives
I/me	want/need	look/see	good, bad
you	like	come	big, little
it	go	play	fast, slow
my/mine	stop	turn	same, different
he	finished/all done/	make	red, blue, green,
she	gone	find	yellow
we	am/is/are	put	happy, sad
they	do	open	pretty
	have	close	old, new
	can	eat	one
	will	drink	
	feel	say/tell	
		read	
		feel	
		colour	
		let's	
		work	

Prepositions	Adverbs	Determiners	Social Words
on, off	more	this	yes
in, out	no/not/don't	that	no
up, down	now	some	thank you
under	here	all	please
to	there		hello
for	away		goodbye
with	again		

NB: The social words can often be indicated in other ways, and so may not need to be included in a communication chart.

Stealers made by a group of AAC users highlighting the shortfalls of a noun-heavy approach.[14] Another sobering YouTube video is called *The Power of Core Vocabulary: Life Saving!*, whereby a young man is able to use core vocabulary to reveal abuse he has experienced.[15]

We need to have a good mix of core and fringe vocabulary. Core vocabulary needs to be easily accessible, so that it can be combined with fringe vocabulary. Core vocabulary might always be consistently placed on various communication charts; it might always be on the left-hand page in a book; or it might be on a fold-out flap. It is useful if the positioning of core words reflects the word order of English, building phrases from left to right. Below is an example of core and fringe vocabulary, as used in an ACE Centre–style communication book.[16] The core words are always on the left-hand page, and fringe words on the right.

We will now look at the different types of AAC. There are slight variations in terminology in the AAC literature when defining no-tech, low-tech, light-tech and

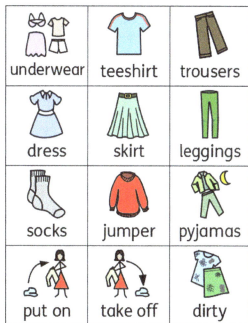

Figure 5.10 Core words and getting dressed

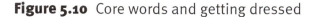

Widgit Symbols © Widgit Software 2002–2017 www.widgit.com

Sample page from a communication book, based on ACE Centre templates,[17] with core words on the left and fringe words on the right.

high-tech. For the purposes of this book, no-tech is AAC that does not require any equipment at all; low-tech is AAC that does not require a battery, and is usually paper-based; light-tech requires a battery but does not have a dynamic screen display; high-tech has a dynamic screen display of text, symbols or images.

No-tech AAC

No-tech AAC does not involve any equipment. It is essentially signs to support spoken language. The main two systems used in the UK are Signalong[18] and Makaton.[19] Makaton has made great strides into popular culture in the last 10 years, largely due to CBeebies' *Something Special* and Mr Tumble. Makaton has become part of most mainstream nurseries and classrooms. It can help all children with their attention and listening and receptive and expressive language development. Makaton signs are especially helpful for children with Down Syndrome, Learning Difficulties and Specific Language Impairment, who need visual representations of language. Signing can also help children with Cerebral Palsy and Autism Spectrum Condition to understand spoken language, though these populations tend to benefit particularly from symbols for expressive language. Unlike British Sign Language (BSL), Makaton and Signalong are always used alongside spoken language, and are not sign languages in their own right. The key words in a sentence are signed, though grammatical elements can be added for some users. Signing can and should be combined with symbol use, as part of multi-modal communication.

Body signing can be used with visually impaired individuals. TaSSeLs: Tactile Signing for Sensory Learners and the Canaan Barrie touch signing systems may be used.[20] A child's signs should then be detailed in a communication passport (see Chapter 13).

Yes/no response

A consistent and clear "yes" or "no" response is arguably the most useful no-tech AAC there is, so that communication partners can quickly check that they are interpreting a message correctly. From early on, it is useful to work on this skill. The form that the yes/no response takes will depend on the physical skills of the individual. The most universally recognised yes/no responses are a nod of the head for "yes" and a shake of the head for "no". These might be reduced to a single movement to reduce the effort. If head movements are too effortful or inaccurate for the individual, then they might sign "yes" and "no", and again these movements might be reduced for the individual's physical skills. A no-tech yes/no is the most preferable, because then the person has a basic communication method wherever they are, with no equipment needed. However, there may be a good reason to use a low-tech solution, like "yes" and "no" wristbands, or light-tech switches (see the following sections).

"I don't know" might be another no-tech gesture or sign to teach, as many questions cannot be answered with a "yes" or "no". This might be a shrug of the shoulders, or it might be a facial expression. "Please" and "thank you" are often taught using signs, because this a quick way of adding these social niceties to an AAC message. How much you prompt "please" and "thank you" depends upon the communication situation. They may be effortful to produce, but they can be important in conveying social competence with unfamiliar partners.

Low-tech AAC

Low-tech AAC does not require a battery. It is usually paper-based, but it does include objects of reference, which are explained shortly. Low-tech should be maintained, even if an AAC user has a high-tech AAC device, because it can be used when a high-tech device is being charged or the environment is not suited to its use.

Low-tech AAC may begin with single photographs or symbols. There used to be an assumption of a hierarchy, with photos being the easiest for young children to understand. However many children are able to begin with symbols, even abstract symbols, which do not look like the thing they represent. What seems to be more important in the learning of a symbol is contingency and consistency: the use of the symbol brings a reward, and/or the caregiver repeatedly matches the symbol to its referent.

Objects of reference

Objects of reference are used with children with Visual Impairment or multiple sensory impairments, who cannot access photos or symbols. An object of reference is an object or a part of an object which stands for an activity or event. For example, a small piece of towel may be used to indicate that it is bath time; a zip may indicate that it is time to get dressed.

The same object of reference is used consistently as a symbol, so that if a plastic cup is used to indicate that it is time for a drink, that cup will never be the one used for drinking. A small number of objects of reference will be selected to reflect the child's activities. These need to be very carefully selected, so that they are accessible: they must have tactile and/or auditory qualities that the child can easily perceive and distinguish. The object of reference will be presented consistently with a verbal label at the start of the activity, to help the child to predict what is going to happen. Objects of reference may then be used for choice-making.

It is suggested that three to six objects of reference are introduced initially. How this vocabulary grows will depend on the response of the child. The collection of objects will be limited by the number of objects that the child can distinguish. Objects of reference may be combined with other AAC, like hand-over-hand or on-the-body signs, high-contrast symbols or Braille.

PECS

PECS,[21] the Picture Exchange Communication System, is a highly structured approach based on ABA, or Applied Behavioural Analysis. Before implementing PECS, practitioners should attend a training course offered by Pyramid, as the structure of PECS and the prompts used are highly prescriptive. PECS aims to move children through the following stages:

1 Make requests through picture exchange. One picture is on offer (e.g. car). The child has to pick up the picture, initially with an adult physical prompt, and give it to another adult. It is then exchanged for a rewarding object.

2 Distance and persistence. The child has to move across a room to get the picture to exchange.

3 Discriminating between pictures. The child has to select between a non-preferred and preferred picture.

4 Sentence structure. The child builds a sentence constructed with "I want" + the picture.

5 Answering questions. The child answers the question "What do you want?"

6 Commenting. However I would argue that this is not commenting; it is answering a question: "What do you see/hear?" The possible answers are "I see a . . .", or "I hear a . . ."

There is now research evidence to show that PECS is effective[22] for building requests for objects (e.g. "I want the ball") but not *social* requests (e.g. "I want a hug", "play with me?"). PECS tends to focus on the behaviour of requesting and answering a question.

For those children with ASC who have very low levels of joint-attention and joint-engagement, it is also worth looking at an approach like *Intensive Interaction*.[23] This approach helps to foster the *fundamentals of communication*, the pre-verbal communication skills that we looked at in Chapter 2. An important element in this approach is that it recognises the shared joy and delight in communication, and that communication involves joint discovery.

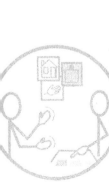

Single symbols

Single symbols may be used to label objects or activities. Choice-making may be introduced, whereby the caregiver holds a symbol in each hand, names them and waits for the child to show a preference. This might include looking or reaching. Later, the child may make a selection from a wider array. The symbols might be reduced in size, and kept on a key-ring or in a container linked to an activity.

Choice-boards

A simple choice-board of two symbols might be introduced, for example "bubbles" or "shaker". The child might look at or reach for a symbol, which would be interpreted as a meaningful choice, even though at first it may not be intentional. This is a "no-fail" choice, where both options are pleasurable. Later, there may be a "preferred" and "non-preferred" symbol (e.g. "ball" and "sock"), to promote conscious choice-making.

Communication boards

Children will quickly need more vocabulary. It is important not to limit the receptive vocabularies of AAC users. Various communication boards should be available to match the different activities with which a child is involved.

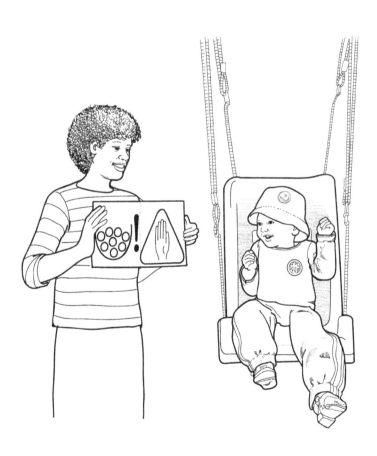

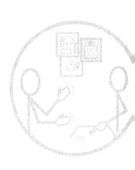

You may want to start with a choice of two symbols, but try to progress to an array of 10–20 symbols. This is provided so the child can visually process this, and can manage to point accurately (see later in the chapter for alternative access to low-tech AAC).

Communication charts should combine "core" vocabulary with "fringe" vocabulary from early on. Examples of early communication charts are shown next. Note the consistent placement of core words, which in this case follows that of the ACE Centre–style of communication book.[24]

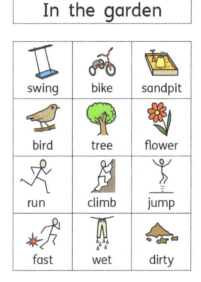

Figure 5.11 Core words in the garden

Widgit Symbols © Widgit Software 2002–2017 www.widgit.com

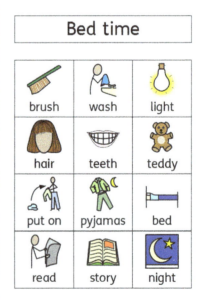

Figure 5.12 Core words bed time

Widgit Symbols © Widgit Software 2002–2017 www.widgit.com

Some suggestions for early communication charts[25]

Table 5.2 Some Suggestions for early communication charts

Getting dressed	Bubble play	Singing songs
Bath time	Ball play	Reading books
Mealtime	Bricks	Simon Says
In the garden	Playdough	Going swimming (laminated!)
At the park	Baby	In the car

The layout of the communication board will need careful consideration depending on the access method and the child's sensory and motor abilities. The size of the grid and the number of cells, the spacing between symbols, and the colour contrasts are all considerations. Input from an Occupational Therapist (OT), Visual Impairment Teacher, Orthoptist or Optometrist is vital if the child has visual impairment or visual processing difficulties. OT input is essential for AAC users with physical impairments, including fine motor difficulties.

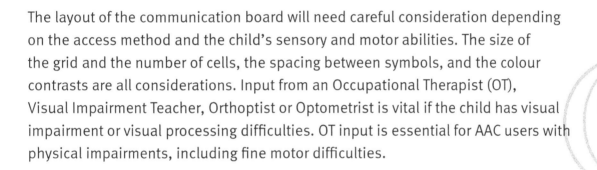

You may feel that pointing to symbols to combine them is not enough, and the child will benefit from physically manipulating single symbols to combine them into phrases. Velcro symbols and a sentence strip may be used. Another option would be to introduce a communication app with a sentence bar (see Chapter 6).

Alphabet charts

We should be aiming for literacy for all of our children (see Chapter 12). Teaching literacy opens up a whole world of creative communication. Symbols will only take you so far: you are limited to the set of symbols that has been chosen for you. Alphabet charts may be combined with core words or quick phrases, as a low-tech backup for high-tech AAC devices. Some AAC practitioners introduce the alphabet to very young children. I would tend to introduce them somewhere around 3 years old, once early communication has been established and a child can attend to an adult's pointing to a picture or symbol.

Figure 5.13 shows examples of low-tech alphabet charts. They may be arranged with an ABC layout, a QWERTY layout, or high-frequency layout. QWERTY is the preference

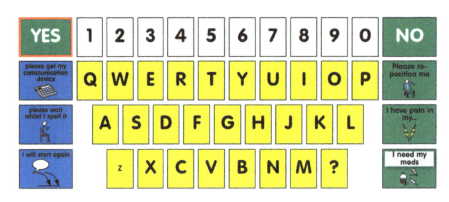

Figure 5.13 Alphabet chart

Alphabet Chart made using MatrixMaker *template, with QWERTY keyboard and WLS.*[26]

for AAC users who will need to use a keyboard for high-tech AAC or curriculum access. The colour contrasts and size will need to be matched to the user.

Alternative access to low-tech AAC

Some children will be able to point to cells on a grid. Children with physical disabilities (e.g. Cerebral Palsy) may need alternative access solutions. These are some examples of alternative access solutions. They will all require the input of an Occupation Therapist.

• Where fist-pointing or eye-pointing is being tried, wide separation of symbols may be needed. Two or four symbols may be located at the corners of the page initially.

• Specialist pointers may be used, to make pointing more accurate. These may be strapped to an arm, hand or head. They may be light or laser pointers.

• Eye-pointing frames, like the E-Tran,[27] made from Perspex, with a hole cut in the centre, and symbols at each of the four corners and possibly in the centre-top and bottom, are useful for a child who is using eye-pointing. The communication partner positions the frame in front of the child to see where their eyes move. Think about the size of the frame: it is tiring for the eyes if the frame is large. An A4 frame made out of laminated card may be more suitable for a child, and is easily transported. A range of frames with different vocabulary can be used.

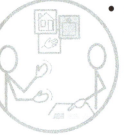

• More complex "coded" access methods can be introduced for able eye-gaze users. Two to six areas of the frame may be colour-coded, and then each symbol in that area is also colour-coded. Coded access allows much more vocabulary to be displayed in one page.

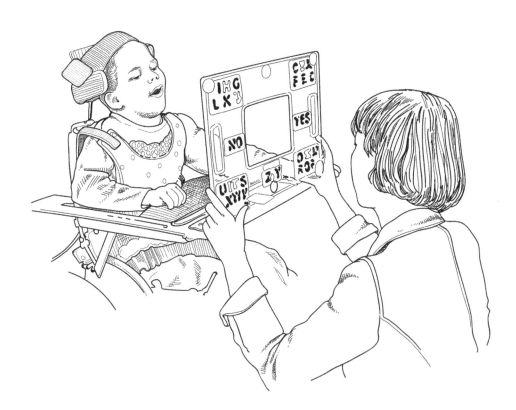

- *Look2Talk*[28] is a very useful eye-pointing resource which makes use of colour-coded access. There is a systematic progression through five stages. Stage 1 introduces two core symbols. Stage 2 allows the combination of the two core symbols, which always stay the same on the left side of the page, with two to four additional fringe symbols to the right of the core. Different pages with different fringe symbols can be added, but the core symbols stay the same. Stage 3 introduces coded access with two colours, which doubles the number of symbols that can be displayed. Further colours are then added to further increase the number of symbol options on a page. Examples based on the *Look2Talk* approach are shown below.

- For children with Visual Impairment, high-contrast symbols may be used, such as high-contrast PCS,[31] which have a black background and bright colours and minimal detail, and Widgit V.I. Symbols,[32] which have stronger colour contrasts, thicker lines and simplified images.

- Laminated sheets can be difficult for children with Visual Impairment or visual processing difficulties to see. Try matte laminate or non-tearable paper instead.

- "Partner-assisted scanning" may be used, whereby an adult will read out the options from a communication chart or book slowly, waiting for a nod or some indication that this is the desired option. Timing is key here: the adult must be sensitive to the child's processing speed to present the options at an

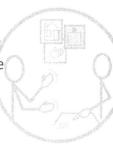

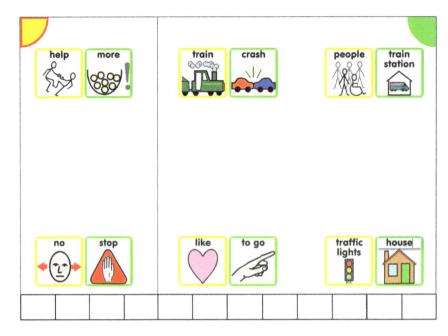

Figure 5.14 Eye pointing 1

Eye-Pointing Colour-coded Communication Chart[29] made using MatrixMaker *template with WLS. To select a symbol, the AAC user first looks to one of the six areas on the page. There are two possible symbols, so the AAC user then looks to the yellow or green areas at the top of the page to indicate which of these two symbols they want. Core vocabulary is on the left, and fringe vocabulary to the right of the line.*

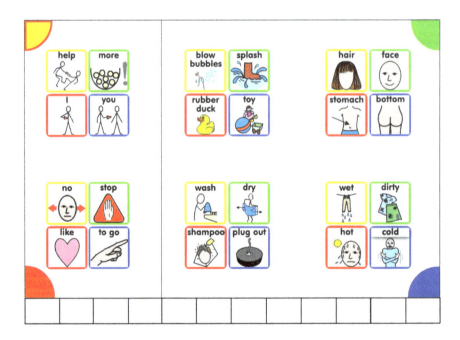

Figure 5.15 Eye pointing 2

Eye-Pointing Colour-coded Communication Chart[30] made using MatrixMaker *template with WLS. To select a symbol, the AAC user first looks to one of the six the areas on the page. There are four possible symbols, so the AAC then looks at one of the four coloured areas in the corners of the page, which corresponds to the symbol they wish to select. Core vocabulary remains on the left, and fringe to the right of the line. Consistent placement of core vocabulary means that the AAC user does not have to re-learn positions when moving up through the stages.*

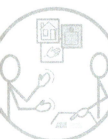

appropriate pace. Partner-assisted scanning might be visual (pointing to symbols as you say the word) or auditory (reading words). Partner assisted auditory scanning communication books might be used for AAC users who have no functional vision. They contain lists of words or phrases, with no symbols.

- For children with social communication difficulties, who may need to exchange a symbol in order to understand that they are requesting, symbols on a grid may be attached with Velcro. It is important that the symbol is replaced in the same position, to promote motor-planning. The base therefore needs to show where symbols should be re-positioned.

Communication books

Move on from charts to a book fairly quickly for a cognitively able child. You can retain the charts in the areas of the house or classroom where that activity takes place. Having a book introduces the child to more vocabulary, and to a way of organising vocabulary. Having a contents page is useful, and tabs so that you can quickly go to the page you need. You may use partner-assisted scanning to offer the child options, or the child might directly access the book by turning pages and pointing to the symbol.

There are various ways of organising a communication book. They include:

- *Activity-Based Communication Book*: Young children tend to need communication books that are organised by activity or situation (e.g. "bath time", "getting dressed", "bubble play", "ball play"). Core and fringe vocabulary would be on the same page, to allow relevant phrases to be constructed. This allows the adult to model language in a given situation, without too many page turns. The pages would reflect the activities of the individual child. The pages are very similar therefore to the activity-based communication charts we have discussed. Core vocabulary should be consistently placed.

- *Category-Based Communication Book*: Vocabulary can be organised in semantic categories (e.g. "People", "Actions", "Places"). The danger with this is that the book becomes a collection of nouns, and so it is important to think about how core and fringe vocabulary might be combined. One solution is to have core words always visible on a fold-out page.

- *Core and Fringe Vocabulary*: The ACE Centre have developed a system of organising core and fringe vocabulary in a activity- or category-based

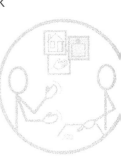

communication book.[33] There are five progressive stages, based on how many core words are used. A child may progress through the levels, but doesn't have to start at Stage 1. This is a tried-and-tested method, and saves professionals from having to re-invent the wheel. Examples are shown below.

- *PODD (Pragmatic Organisation Dynamic Display)*: This system, developed by Gayle Porter,[34] organises an extensive vocabulary according to the pragmatic function (e.g. "I'm telling you something" or "I'm asking a question"). This approach requires adults to be specifically trained in the PODD method of supporting a child. There are many different levels and alternative access versions of PODD, with high-tech versions also available.

Suggested pages for a category-based communication book

(Sub-categories may be added later: these are in brackets.)

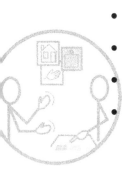

- Help page (e.g. "please get my communication device", "I'm uncomfortable", "I'm unwell")

- People (family, friends, school, therapy, characters, famous people)

- Actions (whole body, work and play, thinking)

- Parts of the body (face, body, medical)

- Clothes (accessories)

- Toys

- Books

- Places (home, community, school, outdoors, UK, world)

- Things (personal equipment, school equipment, bedroom, kitchen, bathroom)

- Food (fruit, vegetables, meals, snacks, puddings, drinks)

- Animals (pets, farm, zoo, woodland, sea, insects)

- Vehicles (land, sea, sky)

- School (literacy, maths, science, art, music, playground)

- Holidays

- Therapy

- Weather

- Time

- Describing words (colours, patterns, shapes, touch, sound)
- Feelings (positive, negative)
- Opinions (positive, negative)
- Questions
- Position words
- I can't find the word, including clues like "it's a bit like . . .", "it's the opposite of . . .", "it looks like . . ." "it's used for . . ." "it starts with . . ."
- Alphabet
- Numbers.

Yes/no solutions

If an AAC user is unable to nod or shake their head or sign "yes" or "no", then it may be useful for them to wear wristbands for "yes" and "no". They would be taught to raise or look at the corresponding wrist. When they are not wearing their wristbands (in bed or in the bath) they might still perform this action for a familiar communication partner to interpret. This is often a better solution than including yes/no symbols in a communication chart or book, because yes/no can be used in any situation, with any other AAC solution, and this strategy often saves time. There is an additional advantage of not needing to take up two cells of every page of symbols with "yes" and "no".

Visual supports

Everyone uses visual support to help them to organise their thoughts and activities. Children with ASC benefit from visual structure,[35] but children with attention and listening difficulties, language impairment and learning difficulties also respond well to this sort of support. These visual supports can be made by hand, or using symbol software such as *Boardmaker*,[36] *InPrint 3*[37] or *Matrix Maker Plus*.[38] Widgit have also produced some very good ready-made resources.[39]

Commonly used visual supports include:

- Now and Next board, to show what has to be done in order to gain a reward.
- Help board, to indicate immediate needs, to avoid meltdowns. For example these might include "it's too loud" or "I don't understand".
- Visual schedule or task breakdown board showing the sequence of actions that need to be completed.

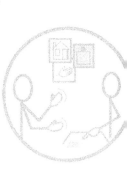

- Visual timetable with removable symbols for the session, including a "surprise!" symbol for changes.

- "I'm working for . . ." board,[40] with 3–5 spaces for stars, and a reward at the end.

- Natural consequences chart, showing what will happen if the desired and non-desired behaviour takes place.

- Opinion charts, such as *Talking Mats*.[41] These provide a visual structure for giving opinions. Velcroed symbols are placed on a board, for example "like", "not sure" and "don't like", along with symbols for different activities. This is very useful for advocacy and EHCPs.[42]

- Communication passports, which give key information about the AAC user's likes and dislikes, communication methods and health needs.[43]

- Credit-card communication cards: a briefer version of a communication passport, which may be especially useful in situations like getting public transport or ordering at a café.

- Topic vocabulary lists, worksheets or mind-maps to accompany a lesson. These might be custom-made using symbol software, or might be purchased.[44]

- Social Stories, to help a child with social communication difficulties to understand behaviour expectations in a specific situation.[45]

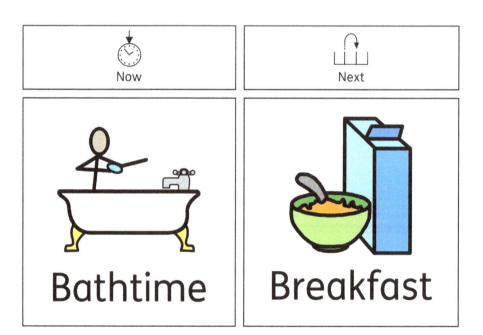

Figure 5.16 Now and next

Widgit Symbols © Widgit Software 2002–2017 www.widgit.com

Now and Next Board[46]

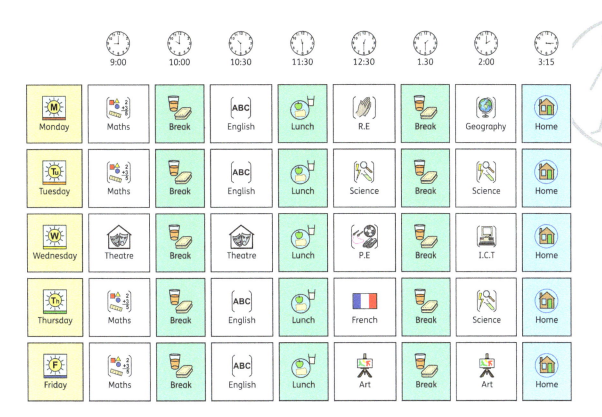

Figure 5.17 Visual timetable

Widgit Symbols © Widgit Software 2002–2017 www.widgit.com

Visual Timetable[47]

My Tasks

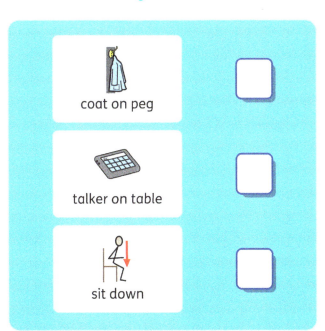

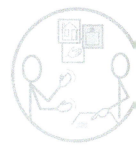

Figure 5.18 Visual schedule

Widgit Symbols © Widgit Software 2002–2017 www.widgit.com

Visual Schedule

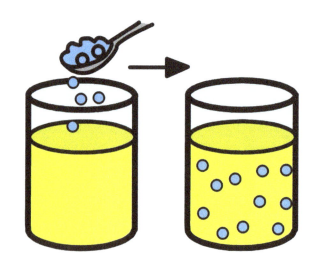

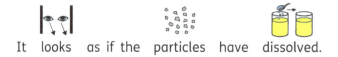

It looks as if the particles have dissolved.

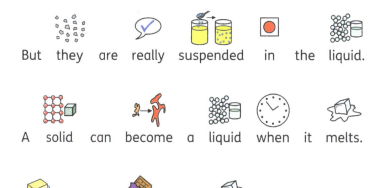

But they are really suspended in the liquid.

A solid can become a liquid when it melts.

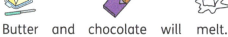

Butter and chocolate will melt.

Figure 5.19 Curriculum worksheet

Widgit Symbols © Widgit Software 2002–2017 www.widgit.com
Curriculum worksheet[48]

Light-tech AAC

Light-tech includes devices with batteries, but where the display of symbols is paper-based, and a change in display requires physical change-over.

Single message devices

These have a single button to press to activate a recorded message. They include BIGmack, Big Point, and Recordable Speech Bubbles. They can be mounted in different ways, including on a wall or in the outdoor area. Some can be adjusted for the amount of pressure or the length of press to activate.

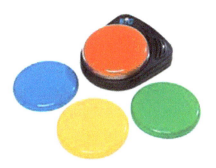

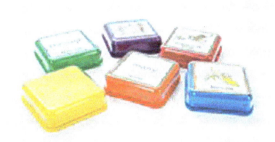

Figure 5.20 BIGmack

BIGmack[49]

Figure 5.21 Big Point

Big Point[50]

For a child with little or no functional speech, these devices introduce the idea of them having a voice, and being able to get someone's attention or make things happen by activating a button and making it speak.

Single message devices are often seen as a first step to high-tech AAC, but may be retained alongside high-tech AAC for specific purposes. For example a button may be placed permanently by a child's bed, on their wheelchair tray or by the toilet, so that they can call for help or give an instruction when other AAC is not available to them.

Some ideas for single-message devices include:[51]

- Say "more bubbles!" when an adult stops blowing them. Alternatives are "more balloon!" (an adult blows up a balloon and lets it go); "more spinner!" (an adult winds up a spinning toy); "more rocket!" (an adult activates a pump to make the rocket fly). Light-up or vibrating toys are also good here.

- Say "go!" in a game of ready-steady-go. The action might be to push the child in a swing; to lift them up high, or let them "fall"; to push them in their buggy or wheelchair.

- Mount a switch by the relevant door saying "I want to go out!" or "I need the toilet!"

- Call the rest of the family to dinner, or tell them when it's bed-time. Give reminders to siblings to "brush teeth" or "get dressed", or to peers at school to "put your coat on".

- Take a message to another person (e.g. "mum says we're late!" or "can we have the register?")

- Say social messages at celebrations, like "Merry Christmas!" or "Happy Birthday!" or "Trick or Treat?"

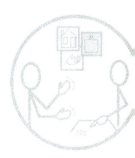

- Ask a question like "what did you do today?" or "what did you do at the weekend?" or "how do you feel today?"

- Take a survey by asking "do you have a pet?" or "what is your favourite book?"

- Mount a switch on a child's wheelchair tray saying "I need my communication book!" or "Beep! Beep!"

- Add a repeated refrain to a story or a song (e.g. "we'll have to go through it!" in *We're Going on a Bear Hunt*).

- Compose a class poem or chant with a repeated refrain every second line (e.g. "and the wind blew cold"). This is surprisingly effective!

Dual- or multi-step message devices

Dual message devices have two buttons with different recorded messages, so that a child can give two different instructions, make a choice, or categorise. For example, they may say "go" or "stop", choose "sand" or "water", or decide that an item is "hard" or "soft".

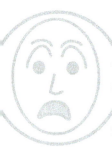

Multi-step devices with sequential messages are also available, so that a child could give a sequence of instructions, or tell a story. Talking photograph albums are another way of recording a number of different messages in a single resource.

Some ideas for dual- and multi-step devices include:

- Say "go" or "stop" to a partner who is carrying out a fun action, like blowing bubbles.

- Say "mine" or "mummy's" when talking treats or toys out of a bag.

- Choose between two activities (e.g. "sand" or "water").

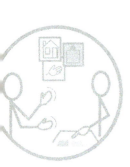

Figure 5.22 BIG Step-by-Step

BIG Step-by-Step[52]

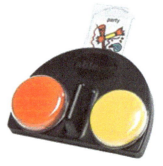

Figure 5.23 iTalk2

iTalk2[53]

- Choose between two items of clothing (e.g. "trousers" or "shorts").

- Choose a partner in a game (e.g. "Dad" or "Hasan").

- Give a command in Simon Says (e.g. "dance", "jump" or "sleep").

- Decide whether something is "yum" or "yuck". This could be extended for other concept work (e.g. "dirty" or "clean", "wet" or "dry", "soft" or "hard").

- Decide where to put items when tidying up or putting shopping away (e.g. "in the fridge" or "in the cupboard").

- Give instructions for a recipe or an experiment (e.g. "add the bicarb to the vinegar", "stand back!").

- Recite a short poem, line by line.

- Say four or five lines in a play script.

- Recite the days of the week, the months of the year, number bonds, or any other rote learning.

- Give clues so that the other person can guess who or what you are describing in a mystery box or bag (e.g. "it is soft", "it's very long", "you wear it on your neck").

- Prepare some interview questions for a special guest.

Multiple overlay devices

These devices have the capacity for an array of a number of symbols, from four symbols per page to 32+. These devices have a number of different levels, usually around five, so that different overlays of symbols can be used. Examples of this type of device include the *Go Talk*[54] range (with 4, 9, 20 and 32 cells per page, and 5 different levels), and the *Super Talker*[55] (with 1, 2, 4 and 8 cells per page, and 8 different levels).

These devices tend to be very robust and long-lived, and can be loaned to many different children in their lifetime. The expense when compared to high-tech tablets at first may appear prohibitive, but high-tech devices tend to have a 3- to 4-year lifetime, whereas these devices can last for 20 years or more. They give a very good indication of whether a voice output device is appealing for a child. For some children, they are also a very good way to prepare them to move from a static display to a dynamic display where they will have to cope with the whole screen changing at the press of one vocabulary cell. By using the multiple overlay device, the child can see the overlays being changed physically from a specific topic that they have chosen (e.g. food) to a new overlay of food + core vocabulary.

Perhaps even more valuable is that some of these devices, like the *Smart/Scan*[56] and the *SuperTalker*, are *switch-accessible*. For children who cannot use direct selection

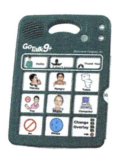

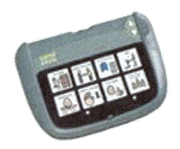

Figure 5.24 GoTalk 9

GoTalk 9[57]

Figure 5.25 SuperTalker

SuperTalker[58]

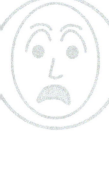

(i.e. they cannot just press a button to activate a cell), using a switch may be their access method. An Occupational Therapist will be able to assess the best switch access method, whether this be a hand, foot, head, chin or other specialist switch. These devices use a scanning pattern, so that they scan through each group, row or column of cells in turn, and the child hits the switch when the desired area or individual cell is reached. The device may be set up to use one switch, in which case the rows and cells will automatically scan at a selected rate, and the child will use their switch to select. The device may also be set up to use two switches, in which case the child will use one switch to move the scanner on, and the other switch to select. A child with Cerebral Palsy can use these light-tech devices to learn scanning patterns that may be used later on with high-tech AAC and curriculum recording software.

Some ideas for using multiple overlay devices include:

- Have pages for different routines in the day (e.g. getting dressed, going out, with a mixture of core and fringe vocabulary on the page).[59]

- Have pages for specific play activities (e.g. doll play, ball play, reading books, singing songs, with a mixture of core and fringe vocabulary).

- Have a car, bus or train journey page for routine journeys where the child might enjoy getting your attention and drawing attention to things you can see.

- Prepare a page for the curriculum topic you are going to be covering this term (e.g. Tudors, Forces). Again include a mixture of core and fringe vocabulary on the page.

- Have pages for key times in the school day (e.g. playtime, register), with the social phrases that are used then (e.g. "do you want to play. . .", "it's your turn"), and so on.

- Have a general chat page (e.g. "my name is. . .", "I have a pet dog", "what do you like to do?").

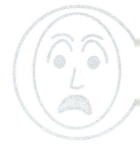

Because these devices have limited levels, you might have to be ruthless and only include key communication situations. You could choose to prioritise core vocabulary and phrases on this device, and have fringe vocabulary on low-tech communication charts or in a book. It is good practice to model combining AAC modes in this way. This light-tech device may only be a temporary resource for this child, but keep all the overlays you make, because they may be used with another child. *MatrixMaker*[60] software has templates for all light-tech devices available in the UK. Overlays can thus be created in a matter of minutes.

Alphabet light tech

The *MegaBee*[61] is a light-tech version of an alphabet E-Tran frame. There is a two-step coding process, so the AAC user first looks at the coloured area, and then at the colour of the letter they need in that area. When the AAC user eye-points their selection, the communication partner clicks the corresponding coloured button at the base of the device. This is easy to do because their thumbs are already positioned there for holding the device. The message then automatically appears

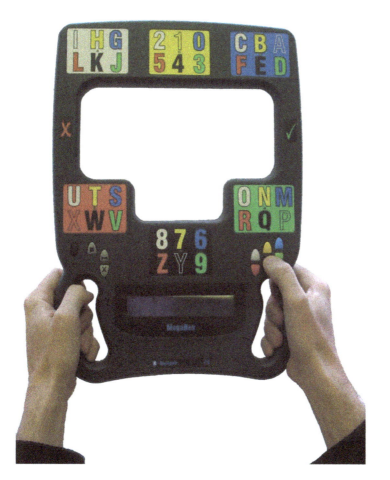

Figure 5.26 The MegaBee

The MegaBee

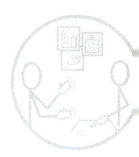

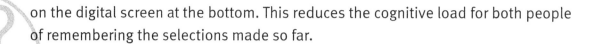

on the digital screen at the bottom. This reduces the cognitive load for both people of remembering the selections made so far.

So far, the no-tech, low-tech and light-tech AAC options may have been implemented without the input of a Specialist AAC Hub Centre.

In the next chapter, we will examine high-tech AAC. If this is the practitioner's first experience of high-tech AAC, or the individual they are working with has complex AAC needs, this next stage is likely to involve a referral to a Specialised AAC Assessment Hub Centre.

You are not alone!

Notes

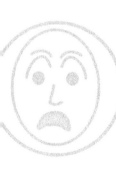

1 Wilkinson, K., Light, J. and Drager, K. (2012) Considerations for the composition of visual scene displays: potential contributions of information from visual and cognitive sciences. *Augmentative and Alternative Communication*, 28(3), 137–147.
2 http://boardmakeronline.com and http://inclusive.co.uk.
3 Andy Bondy, PhD and Lori Frost, MS, CCC-SLP at Pyramid Educational Consultants (www.pecs.com).
4 www.widgit.com.
5 http://boardmakeronline.com and http://inclusive.co.uk.
6 http://inclusive.co.uk.
7 Banajee, M., DiCarlo, C. and Stricklin, S. (2009) Core vocabulary determination for toddlers. *Augmentative and Alternative Communication*, 19(2), 67–73; Fallon, K., Light, J. and Paige, T. (2001) Enhancing vocabulary selection for preschoolers who require Augmentative and Alternative Communication (AAC). *American Journal of Speech-Language Pathology*, 10, 81–94.
8 Lee, Y. M., Kim, Y. T. and Park, E. H. (2005) A preliminary study for the core and fringe AAC vocabulary used by elementary school students. *Communication Sciences and Disorders*, 10(1), 134–152.
9 Lee, Y. M., Kim, Y. T. and Park, E. H. (2005) A preliminary study for the core and fringe AAC vocabulary used by elementary school students. *Communication Sciences and Disorders*, 10(1), 134–152.
10 Made using *InPrint:3*.
11 Made using *InPrint:3*.
12 http://acecentre.org.uk/symbol-charts.
13 Adapted from http://aaclanguagelab.com/files/100highfrequencycorewords2.pdf.
14 https://www.youtube.com/watch?v=Vib2__BDCXc.
15 https://www.youtube.com/watch?v=QqfVAPuGzpl.
16 Latham, C. (2004) *Developing and Using a Communication Book*. Oxford: ACE Centre Advisory Trust.

17 Ibid.

18 http://signalong.org.uk.

19 http://makaton.org.

20 http://sensorysupportservice.org.uk/wp-content/uploads/2014/10/Body-Signing-Special-School-Inset-Compatibility-Mode.pdf.

21 http://pecs-unitedkingdom.com.

22 Gordon, K., Pasco, G., McElduff, F., Wade, A., Howlin, P. and Charman, T. (2011) A communication-based intervention for nonverbal children with autism: What changes? Who benefits? *Journal of Consulting and Clinical Psychology*, 79(4), 447–457.

23 Hewett, D., Barber, M. and Firth, G. (2011) *The Intensive Interaction Handbook*. London: Sage.

24 Latham, C. (2004) *Developing and Using a Communication Book*. Oxford: ACE Centre Advisory Trust.

25 These can also be used with Multiple Overlay Devices (light-tech AAC, later on in this chapter) and Visual Scene Displays (high-tech AAC in Chapter 6).

26 http://inclusive.co.uk.

27 http://liberator.co.uk.

28 Latham, C. and Buckley, K. (2008) *Look2Talk Guidebook*. Oxford: ACE Centre Advisory Trust.

29 Based on Latham, C. and Buckley, K. (2008) *Look2Learn Communication Book*. Oxford: ACE Centre Advisory Trust.

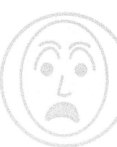

30 Ibid.

31 http://mayer-johnson.com.

32 www.widgit.com.

33 Latham, C. (2004) *Developing and Using a Communication Book*. Oxford: ACE Centre Advisory Trust.

34 http://novita.org.au.

35 See http://autism.org.uk for more information.

36 http://boardmakeronline.com, http://inclusive.co.uk or http://toby-churchill.com.

37 www.widgit.com.

38 http://inclusive.co.uk.

39 www.widgit.com/resources/curriculum.

40 http://educateautism.com offers free downloads.

41 http://talkingmats.com.

42 Education, Health and Care Plans. See Chapter 16.

43 http://communicationpassports.org.uk.

44 www.widgit.com has a range of symbol resource packs around curriculum topics.

45 http://carolgraysocialstories.com.

46 Widgit.com Autism Support Pack.

47 Widgit.com Autism Support Pack.

48 Widgit.com Curriculum Symbol Resource Pack.

49 http://inclusive.co.uk.

50 Ibid.

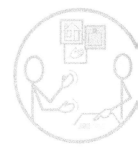

51 See also *101 Ideas for Using the BIGmack*, http://ablenetinc.com/downloads/dl/file/id/32/product/31/101_ideas_single_message_sgd.pdf.

52 http://inclusive.co.uk.

53 Ibid.

54 Ibid.

55 Ibid.

56 Ibid.

57 Ibid.

58 Ibid.

59 See the section on low-tech AAC: "Some Suggestions for Communication Charts" on p. XX in *this chapter (5)*.

60 http://inclusive.co.uk.

61 http://liberator.co.uk.

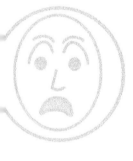

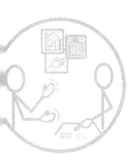

Chapter 6

High-tech AAC

This is where you might get scared. This chapter may look completely overwhelming, but you are never alone in this. This is where your Regional Specialised AAC Assessment Hub Service comes in.

Hub and Spoke model

The *Hub and Spoke* model of AAC commissioning from NHS England was introduced in 2015. This provision model sets out how local and regional services should work together to provide AAC support for those with the most complex communication needs.

Scotland, Wales and Northern Ireland also have regional AAC Assessment Centres, though the funding arrangements are slightly different. An up-to-date list of regional AAC Assessment Centres and current best practice guidelines are available from Communication Matters.[1] *The Right to Speak*[2] is a document setting out the plan for AAC services in Scotland. As yet there is no equivalent for Wales or Northern Ireland.

A *Decision Tree* is shown in Chapter 10. The decision tree will help clinicians in England to decide whether referral to a Hub is indicated, or whether their AAC needs can be met by the Spoke Service. Professionals in Scotland, Wales and Northern Ireland are advised to check the referral criteria to their regional or national AAC services.

Around 90% of the AAC population require Local Spoke AAC Services alone. Ten per cent will require Regional Specialised Hub AAC Services.[3]

The Hub and Spoke (or Regional and Local) services are commissioned to work closely together to ensure the best pathway for AAC users with the most complex needs. Some roles and responsibilities are negotiable: some Spoke Services will have the necessary expertise within their team, where others will need to draw on the resources of the Hub Service. The Hub and Spoke services are commissioned to work together to support individuals, to provide the necessary AAC training and support to families, schools and other partners, and to maintain and update equipment as necessary. Loan banks of equipment are available to Spoke services so that they can trial AAC solutions. This can inform whether referral to the Hub is indicated.

Hubs often offer *one-off consultations* for clients, their families and the professionals working with them. These consultations involve all relevant people coming together

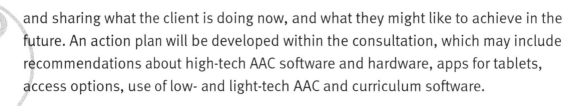

and sharing what the client is doing now, and what they might like to achieve in the future. An action plan will be developed within the consultation, which may include recommendations about high-tech AAC software and hardware, apps for tablets, access options, use of low- and light-tech AAC and curriculum software.

Some clients will require *full assessment* for a bespoke AAC solution, which may involve a mainstream or dedicated AAC device, specialist software, and/or bespoke access and mounting. It is recommended that you discuss a possible referral to the AAC Hub if you are inexperienced in referring.

Referral criteria to a Specialised AAC Assessment Hub

See Chapter 10 for the referral criteria and *Decision Tree*, designed to help in the decision-making process when considering referral to a Hub.

If an individual does not meet the criteria for a Regional Hub Service referral, then they will continue to be managed by the Local Spoke Service.

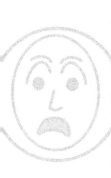

The following sections are intended to be a rough guide to communication apps, specialist software and hardware. The list is not comprehensive. It reflects the most commonly used solutions. It would take many more pages to include all available solutions. The main features of each are discussed, but more information is available on the relevant website for each product. The information included is accurate at the time of writing. New products are constantly being developed, so refer to suppliers' websites.

Don't panic!

You are not expected to memorise these products and their features: that is for your local AAC Hub! I include this information because you may have used or heard of some of the products, and may be interested in learning about others. Please consult your regional AAC Hub if you have questions about which product to purchase.

Voice amplifiers

This is an option for people who have a very quiet voice, perhaps because of insufficient breath support, or because of damage to their larynx after intubation. Voice amplifiers are small and lightweight, clipping on to clothing. Amplification of breath sounds can be a problem, but this can be remedied by using a microphone windshield, by positioning the microphone differently, or by using a microphone that reduces the frequencies associated with breathing sounds. Mobile phone and PC compatibility are recommended features.

Communication apps

Over the last five years, there have been a plethora of communication apps available through the *Apple iTunes App Store* for Apple devices. More recently, *Google Play* have begun to release apps for Android devices. So far these have been of relatively poor quality, and the diversity of Android tablets means that some devices simply do not have the processing power to run these apps. In the list that follows, iOS (Apple) apps predominate, but the Android market is likely to catch up over time, and I expect that in time these apps will be available in both formats. CALL Scotland produce up-to-date information on apps for Android and Apple devices on their website.[4]

Complete vocabulary or specific functions?

Some communication apps are for specific communication functions. For example, *Talking Mats* is for giving opinions and *PECS* is for requesting. Other communication apps offer a complete vocabulary package which can be used for the full range of communication purposes. Some communication apps can be highly personalised, whilst others are only available as a "lite" version on the app, and the full version must be purchased for a PC or communication device. The lite versions fill a market niche, bridging the gap between light-tech and specialist high-tech, and are extremely valuable for trialling with children who may be ready for high-tech AAC.

For communication or word processing?

The apps at the top of the table are for spoken communication. Those that are essentially word processors, for creating written texts (though this may sometimes be used for spoken communication too) are specified.

Display options

The communication apps that have a full vocabulary package fall broadly into three display designs. These may be used in combination:

- *Visual Scene Displays* of photographs of communication situations with *hotspots* programmed with sounds, spoken words or phrases and written words. These tend to engage early communicators, and relate the vocabulary to a child's real-life communication environments. There is an increasing body of research evidence surrounding Visual Scene Displays.[5]

- *Symbol Grids*, in which symbols are organised into pages of grids of symbols, by semantic category or pragmatic function. These typically have a *sentence bar* at the top of the screen, so that a sequence of symbols can be selected to make a phrase or sentence.

- *Text-to-Speech*, in which cells in a grid are populated by written words or phrases, or there is an onscreen keyboard allowing the user to type, and possibly use

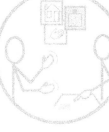

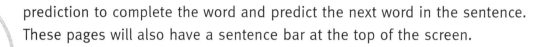

prediction to complete the word and predict the next word in the sentence. These pages will also have a sentence bar at the top of the screen.

Voice options

Communication apps nearly all have voice output. There are various types of voice output:

- *Recorded speech*. This is useful for adding sound effects to some symbols or to Visual Scene Displays, but you would not want to have to programme a whole app with recorded speech. Therefore apps generally come pre-programmed with one of the two following.

- *Synthesised speech*. This is computerised speech, using an artificial voice, and so can sound a little unnatural. The quality of synthesised speech has improved dramatically in the last few years.

- *Digitised speech*. This is recorded human speech. Thousands of words and phrases will have been recorded, to produce an effect that is more natural-sounding. Standard voices are available for male and female, adult and child. Most communication apps and software use this option, with *Acapela* and *Nuance* voices commonly being used. Additional voices may be available for a given app or piece of software, including those with regional accents.

- *Voice-banking*. This is an option for adults with progressive degenerative conditions.[6] They can record their own voice, before it deteriorates, to use later on a communication device. The individual will need to record around 1,600 sentences, which will take 8 hours or longer.

Switch accessibility

Many apps can now be made switch-accessible. For iPads this can be enabled by using the iPad iOS Switch Control feature in the iPad Settings and a compatible switch interface (e.g. *APPlicator* or *iSwitch*).[7] For Android devices, switches can be connected using a USB or Bluetooth connection. Preferences for switch-scanning can then be set up in settings. It is possible to enable one or two switches, with various scanning patterns, sound effects or speech with scanning. The degree to which you can personalise the switch settings varies with the type of switch you are using. This is worth investigating thoroughly before an app is purchased. It is recommended that you contact the app developer when looking at bespoke access. It is also worth knowing that all apps can be made switch-accessible to a degree. This works best for cause-and-effect games. "Recipes" can be made: activating the switch will make a predetermined action occur (e.g. as if you have swiped or pressed the screen). Inclusive.co.uk have some very good webinars on how to use switches with iPads and Android devices.[8]

Table 6.1 Apps

Name of App	Cost	Description
PECS	£5.99–£79.99	Designed to look like low-tech PECS books. PECS III focuses on discrimination between symbols. PECS IV+ includes sentence starters and the sentence strip, and is intended for learners who have mastered phases I to IV of PECS. Photos can be uploaded. Uses Pics for PECS symbols. The voice can be turned on or off.
Snap Scene	Free–£39.99	Visual Scene Display communication app. The free version is limited to 10 preloaded scenes, but the full version allows uploading of personalised scenes. Insert sounds and words into hot spots on the visual display. No symbols. A companion app, Pathways, offers tips and videos on how to use visual scene displays in play situations. Available for Windows, Android and Apple devices.
ChatAble	£79.99	Visual Scene Display, symbol-based, or hybrid communication app. Pages can be printed and emailed. Emoticon sound effects. Includes access to social media, and so is a good option for adults. Wide range of voices, including a voice-banking option for users with degenerative conditions. Handwriting and keyboard input options. iOS switch control. WLS.

(*Continued*)

Table 6.1 (Continued)

Name of App	Cost	Description
Scene and Heard	£199.99	Visual Scene Display. Upload photographs of communication situations to create visual scene displays and to link scenes. Insert symbols, video or audio clips into hotspots on the display. Create printable pages in a communication book, visual tasks and timetables. iOS switch control. WLS.
Clicker Communicator	£199.99	Symbol-based communication app. Vocabulary packages with three levels, which can be customised. Additional pages can be downloaded for free. Visually clear layout, with a good balance of core and fringe vocabulary. Switch-accessible. "SuperKeys" feature increases the size of a selected cell set. There is also a good keyboard with symbolised prediction. Switch-accessible. SymbolStix, WLS or PCS versions are available.
GridPlayer	Free version; can also be used with Grid 3 packages if this has been purchased.	Symbol- or text-based communication app. Two symbol-based vocabulary packages, plus Talking Photos and Text Talker Phrasebook. These can't be customised in the free app. Visually clear layout, with a mix of core and fringe vocabulary on each topic page. Comes with WLS. Like Clicker Communicator, this is a good communication app to try with students who have not used a VOCA before. They may progress to Grid 3, a more extensive software package for a range of devices, which costs £480. There is no onscreen keyboard with the app. Several languages are available. WLS.

Name of App	Cost	Description
TD Compass	£139.99	Visual Scene Display, symbol- or text-based communication app. Complete vocabulary packages with multiple levels and various display options. "NavBar" navigation, quick fire phrases and behavioural supports, alongside more traditional grids and keyboard options. Personalisation will enhance this package. Switch-accessible. Available for Android and iPad. PCS.
Widgit Go	Free–£54.99	Symbol-based learning and communication app. Not a complete vocabulary package, but an app that enables you to create communication grids and printable resources. The free version comes with 14 example activities, whilst the full version allows editing. It is more curriculum-focused than other communication apps. No onscreen keyboard. Available for Android and iPad. WLS.
Proloquo2Go	£199.99	Symbol-based communication app. Extensive package with three vocabulary levels (each with extra vocabulary that can be easily imported) and multiple layout options. There is an extensive range of vocabulary pages, and these can be personalised further. There is a consistent layout of core vocabulary on every page: helpful for motor-planning. There are grammar options for word endings for higher-level language-learning. iOS switch control. SymbolStix.

(*Continued*)

Table 6.1 (Continued)

Name of App	Cost	Description
Proloquo4Text		Text-to-speech communication app, with keyboard, stored words and phrases. Self-learning word prediction. Many different voices and languages available. Social media compatible. Split view mode to view two apps at the same time. iOS switch control.
Predictable	£119.99	Text-to-speech communication app with "intelligent word prediction", which learns the user's patterns. QWERTY, ABC or high-frequency keyboard options. Allows voice-banking, for users with degenerative conditions, who would prefer to have their own voice rather than a synthesised voice. iOS switch control.
Co:Writer Universal	£14.99	Developed as a typing app, but can also be used as a text-to-speech communication app. Word prediction for phonetic and personal spellings. Four million topic-specific vocabularies can be accessed.
SuperKeys	£12.99	This app works with your onscreen keyboard to enlarge the group of six to seven keys on the keyboard. Word prediction too.

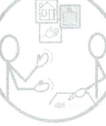

Name of App	Cost	Description
Write ONLINE **Write Online**	£24.99	Typing app, which can also be used as a text-to-speech communication app. Word prediction. Word bars (similar to word banks) can be created for different topics, and words can be organised with alphabetical tabs. Spell check is also speech supported. This app is currently being updated and will be released with a new name shortly. See cricksoft.com for details.
Clicker Sentences Clicker Connect Clicker Books Clicker Docs **Clicker apps**	£31.99	This series of apps is based on Clicker 7 curriculum software. They allow children to create pieces of work using words and pictures. The text can be spoken, enabling the child to check and appreciate their work. Clicker Sentences allows children to build sentences from words that are provided. Clicker Connect involves selecting the next word from a choice. Clicker Books allows the child to make a talking book. Clicker Docs introduces word banks and word prediction to increase the rate of word processing. SuperKeys is also included. These apps can be personalised for spelling, speech, prediction and appearance. Thousands of ready-made online grids can be downloaded. This is a fantastic resource for written recording (as opposed to a vocabulary package for spoken communication).

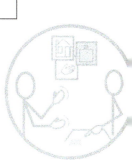

Specialist software for high-tech vocabulary packages

These are the more bespoke solutions that are likely to be recommended by Regional AAC Assessment Hubs following a full assessment. Local Spoke Services are not expected to have an in-depth knowledge of these packages, but they are included for the reader's interest.

These packages are generally designed to be suitable for users with complex access needs, including switch-scanning, eye-gaze and head-mouse. The following is not an exhaustive list of vocabulary packages used in the UK. New products are being released all the time. For up-to-date information, visit the suppliers' websites.

Table 6.2 Examples of Vocabulary Packages: Grid 3

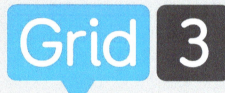

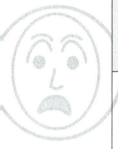

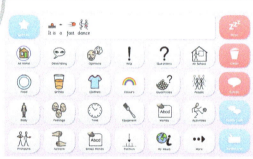

Symbol Talker

Widgit Symbols © Widgit Software 2002–2017 www.widgit.com

- Symbol Talker offers a progressive series of category-based vocabulary packages.
- There is a combination of core and fringe vocabulary on each page.
- Symbol Talker A has the capacity to combine two symbols in a phrase.
- Symbol Taker B has the capacity to combine three symbols in a phrase.
- Symbol Talker C has more core vocabulary on each page, allowing phrases of four symbols.
- Symbol Talker D has smart grammar, allowing grammatically correct sentences to be created.
- Includes an onscreen keyboard with symbolised prediction.
- WLS.

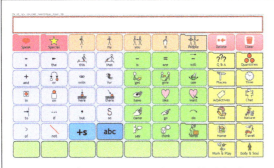

Talkative (currently only available in Grid 2, but will be updated for Grid 3)

Widgit Symbols © Widgit Software 2002–2017 www.widgit.com

- A very extensive package for children and adults.
- Clear visual layout, with core vocabulary on the home page and topic pages to the right.
- Within each topic page, there are many sub-categories, and quick-chat cells at the bottom of the page.
- Predictive grammar from the home page, to allow the user to create grammatically correct sentences.
- Includes an onscreen keyboard with symbolised prediction.
- WLS.

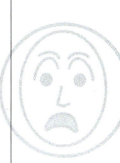

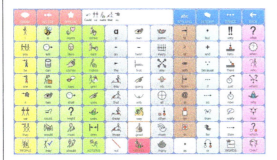

Beeline

Widgit Symbols © Widgit Software 2002–2017 www.widgit.com

- This package has lots of vocabulary on very few pages, so that there is reduced need for navigation between pages.
- This is good for users who like to be able to see what is in the vocabulary package, and don't want frequent page changes.
- It has a clear visual layout, with colour-coded columns.
- Includes an onscreen keyboard with symbolised prediction.
- WLS.

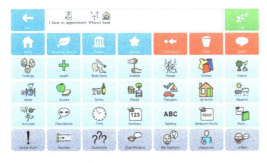

Vocabulary for Life

Widgit Symbols © Widgit Software 2002–2017 www.widgit.com

- This package is designed for older teens and young adults.
- It focuses on social contexts, and offers pre-stored phrases for work and social situations.
- This package is good for users who may struggle with a more creative, language-generating package.
- Includes "adult" language (swear words).
- WLS.

(Continued)

Table 6.2 (Continued)

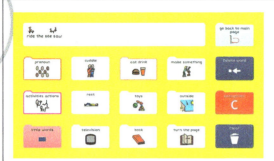

PODD Pragmatic Organisation Dynamic Display

The Picture Communication Symbols © 1981–2017 by Tobii Dynavox. All Rights Reserved Worldwide. Used with permission.

- This vocabulary package replicates low-tech PODD, using a pragmatic organisation of vocabulary.
- Extensive vocabulary.
- Range of pragmatic functions.
- The system requires supportive communication partners to learn the PODD navigation.
- PCS.

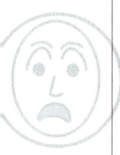

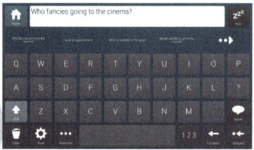

Fast Talker

- A text-based package.
- A range of keyboard options are available, with various colours and layouts.
- The package uses Swift Key prediction, which learns the user's spelling patterns.
- The package also uses location-relevant phrases, so that the user can ask for coffee as soon as they enter the coffee shop.
- Text.
- All of the above Grid 3 packages link to other computer applications, including social media and environmental control.

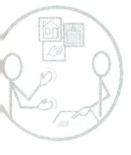

Table 6.3 Examples of Vocabulary Packages: Techcess

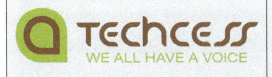

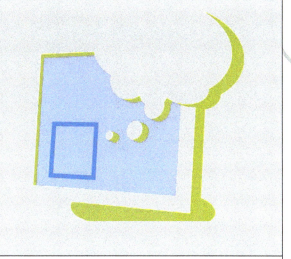

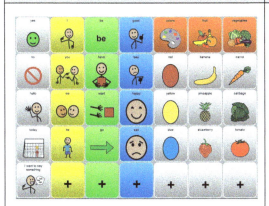

Mind Express 4

SymbolStix®, Copyright 2017, SymbolStix, LLC. All rights reserved. Used with permission.

- Visually attractive platform from which you can create a vocabulary package, with pleasing colour-coded layout.
- Built-in grammar module automatically conjugates verbs
- "Dynamic lists" feature, so that only the fringe words on a page will change as you scroll through a vocabulary list: the rest of the page will stay the same.
- Other applications can be opened in the "Dynamic Lists" part of the screen, allowing for simultaneous core communication alongside a book or movie.
- The package includes a word processor allowing lists and letters to be written.
- The keyboard can be used in other applications on the device.
- SymbolStix, WLS, PCS and others.
- Other vocabulary packages are available which use the Mind Express platform: see *Techcess* website.[9]

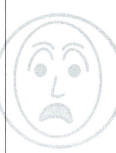

(*Continued*)

Table 6.3 (Continued)

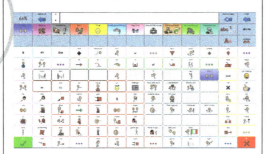

Score

- High-tech version of *Cologne Boards and Binder*, a research-based language programme.
- Consistent placement of core vocabulary with "Dynamic lists" feature for fringe vocabulary.
- Other applications can be opened in the "Dynamic Lists" part of the screen, allowing for simultaneous core communication alongside a book or movie.
- This programme requires the teaching of syntax and grammar: users select grammatical features such as verb tenses as they build correct sentences. It is therefore less suited to users with complex access needs, as more key-presses are needed.
- However, this programme does promote a high level of language and literacy competence.
- The number of cells per page is very high, making it less suitable for eye-gaze users, those with visual processing difficulties and devices with smaller screens.
- SymbolStix.

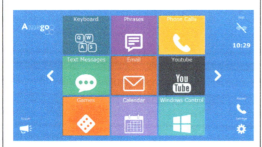

Amego

- A text-based package.
- Visually attractive and contemporary.
- Links to other applications including social media, which can easily be selected or deselected for the user.
- The package adapts to the access method, for example by generating a rest cell on each page for an eye-gaze user.
- Users can easily swap from one access method to another.
- Users can easily change colour-schemes to adapt to lighting conditions.

Table 6.4 Examples of Vocabulary Packages: Compass

tobii dynavox

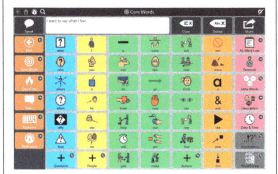

Core First (Snap)

Used with permission ©1981–2017 Tobii Dynavox. All Rights Reserved Worldwide.

- Core First is a vocabulary package with two options: the Fitzgerald Key for symbols, or Keyboard Core.
- Quickfire phrases and behaviour supports within the same package.
- New Pageset Wizard helps to find the right level of vocabulary for the user.
- PCS, with high-contrast and thin-line options.

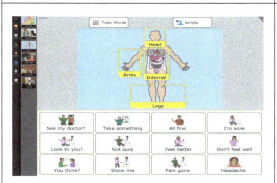

Compass showing Visual Scene Display and NavBar

Used with permission ©1981–2017 Tobii Dynavox. All Rights Reserved Worldwide.

- Visual Scene Display, symbol- and text-based communication packages with many levels.
- Visual Scene Displays can be personalised with photographs of the user and their friends/family in different communication situations. Hotspots then link to additional pages of vocabulary.
- The NavBar to the left of the screen allows users to scroll through the other pages easily. This cannot be switched off, and might be distracting for some users.
- Quickfire phrases and behaviour supports within the same package.
- New Pageset Wizard helps to find the right level of vocabulary for the user.
- PCS, with high-contrast and thin-line options.

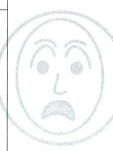

(Continued)

Table 6.4 (Continued)

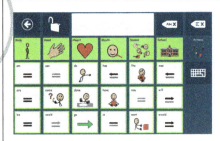

Communicator 5

SymbolStix®, Copyright 2017, SymbolStix, LLC. All rights reserved. Used with permission.

Used with permission ©1981–2017 Tobii Dynavox. All Rights Reserved Worldwide.

- Visual Scene Display, symbol- and text-based communication package with many levels.
- Dwell-free typing for eye-gaze users to enhance speed.
- The same keyboard can be used in other Windows applications.
- Users can switch easily between access methods.
- Links to other computer applications such as social media, and environmental control.
- PCS and SymbolStix.

Table 6.5 Examples of Vocabulary Packages: Saltillo

Saltillo

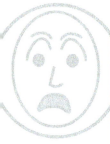

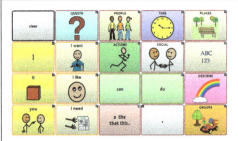

Word Power Simply

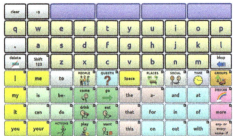

Word Power

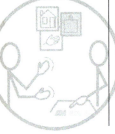

- The Chat software from Saltillo is only available on the NOVAchat and Chat Fusion range of communication devices.
- Both symbol- and text-based packages are available, with many levels.
- The software predicts which concepts you might need next, to improve the flow of conversation.
- Requires a cognitively able user, who has good receptive language and can hold their message in their mind and not get distracted by the changing options on display.
- Not suitable for users who rely on motor-planning to quickly find vocabulary.
- The spelling is American, and words are often abbreviated, which is not helpful for developing literacy.

	<ul><li>The software is only available on dedicated devices which cannot run other applications, so there are no environmental controls or access to social media.</li><li>However, many children benefit from having a dedicated communication device, so that they don't become distracted by other apps.</li><li>The devices are very rugged and reliable.</li><li>SymbolStix and text. PCS can be purchased.</li></ul>

Table 6.6 Examples of Vocabulary Packages available from Liberator UK

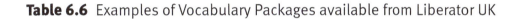

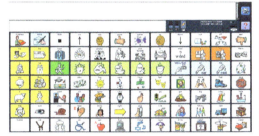

LAMP
(Unity/Minspeak)

- LAMP, or Language Acquisition through Motor Planning, is a system designed for children with ASC. Children learn a consistent motor pattern for accessing a word, often with two-button presses per word.
- LAMP is based on the Unity Language System, with "multi-meaning icons". Two icons are combined to create a word (icon-sequencing). This reduces the number of pages of vocabulary.
- The motor planning sequence for each word is taught through modelling in everyday communication situations.
- The concept of LAMP can be challenging for families.
- LAMP training courses are available. Support from a LAMP-certified professional is recommended.
- Minsymbols.

(*Continued*)

Table 6.6 (Continued)

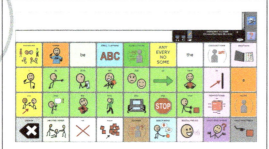 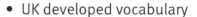 **easyChat** *SymbolStix®, Copyright 2017, SymbolStix, LLC. All rights reserved. Used with permission.*	• UK developed vocabulary • easyChat Phrases, Core, Spell and Word versions are available, offering easy access to core and fringe vocabulary, quick phrases, spelling and word prediction. • Word classes are colour-coded according to the Fitzgerald key. • Grammar support. • A variety of grid sizes. • Other mainstream computer applications can be combined with this package, including Word. • Mobile phone commands and environmental controls are also included, with easy toggling between applications. • SymbolStix.
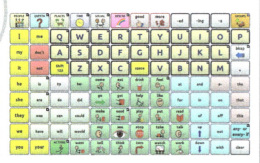 **WordPower and Picture WordPower**	• Symbol- or text-based system. • Combines core and fringe vocabulary with spelling and word prediction. • A variety of grid sizes: 45, 60, 84 or 144 keys. • Fully customizable. • Available on dedicated devices only. • PCS and Minsymbols.
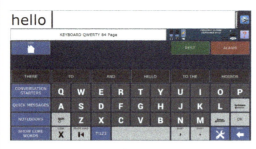 **Essence**	• Text-based programme for users with good literacy skills. Pre-stored phrases and word prediction. • A variety of keyboard options are available. • Word processing, email and internet access. • Environmental controls. • A visually attractive package.

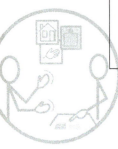

Curriculum software for recording written work

So far we have talked about software to help an individual use the spoken word. There is also software available to help an individual use the written word. Symbols are a low-tech way of helping children read a written word. We advise that for children, symbols are accompanied by the written word, just as Makaton and Signalong signs are always accompanied by the spoken word. For children, symbols can be a way in to literacy, and some children will progress from a symbol-based vocabulary to a text-based vocabulary. If *learning to read* is the activity, then text may be used without symbols, as symbols can distract a child who is learning to decode. If *communication* is the activity, then symbols can be used with text.

A light-tech device that helps with reading words is a talking pen (e.g. *PENpal*). When held over a written word on an enabled resource, this device speaks the word aloud.

A high-tech solution for reading is text-to-speech software. This is fairly widely available and some software is free. CALL Scotland have free text-to-speech reading software called *WordTalk* for Windows available on their website. Others are available, including *Adobe Read Out Loud* and *Natural Reader*.[10] Regional accents are becoming more widely available. These pieces of software tend to operate alongside other mainstream computer software.

The following table includes commonly used software to support curriculum learning and word processing.

Table 6.7 Software

Software	Description
Choose It! Maker[11]	This includes a huge range of curriculum resources for a range of subjects. They use multiple-choice questions to support learning in finely graded steps. Switch-accessible. See Chapter 12 for more information.
SymWriter 2[12]	This is a symbol-supported word processor, allowing the user to generate a range of different documents. This has text-to-speech, symbolised spelling prediction and smart symbolising word prediction, whereby the software predicts the correct symbol where there may be multiple meanings. Switch-accessible. WLS.

(*Continued*)

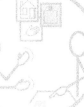

Table 6.7 (Continued)

Software	Description
Boardmaker Online and Studio[13]	This allows the creation of activities and multi-page documents online or to print. CVC Word Builder, with text-to-speech reading, is especially recommended. Direct touch users can access interactive activities on an iPad as well as Windows or Mac devices. Switch-scanning and eye-gaze accessible.
Clicker 7[14]	This is an extensive literacy software package, which allows a child to record their learning across the curriculum. It offers symbolised or text-only word processing for a variety of documents, including books, mind-maps and worksheets. There is an extensive bank of pictures, and additional pictures and word banks can be easily imported into a document. Clicker includes personalised word prediction for typing, text-to-speech reading, and *SuperKeys* function whereby a smaller number of buttons are enlarged on the screen for easy access. A user may use a variety of access methods, including eye-gaze. See Chapter 12 for more information about using Clicker to support Curriculum access and written recording. Switch- and eye-gaze accessible. WLS. PCS and SymbolStix can also be added.
Write Online[15]	This offers age-appropriate text-based word processing for secondary school students. It has personalised word prediction, text-to-speech reading, word bars (similar to word banks in Clicker), writing frames and mind-mapping. Word bars for all curriculum topics can be imported for free. Links to relevant websites for research can be added. Switch-accessible. Requires an internet connection. Text-based. This software is currently being updated and will be released with a new name shortly. See http://cricksoft.com for details.
Penfriend[16]	This assists with the physical demands of typing. It provides an onscreen keyboard with word prediction, for spelling and grammar, and with access to a thesaurus and dictionaries. There is text-to-speech feedback (screen reading), including speaking phonemes. This software is suitable for able AAC users. Specialist lexicons (similar to word banks) can be added (e.g. scientific English, business English). Therefore this is suited to AAC users at University and in the workplace. Switch-accessible.

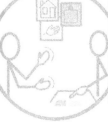

The communication device

So far we have talked about software options. Now we will talk about the hardware: the high-tech communication device itself. Like the specialist software, the Regional AAC Hub Services are expected to have detailed knowledge of these devices, rather than Local Spoke Services. The table that follows, like those earlier, is for the reader's interest only, and does not have to be memorised!

Some considerations when choosing a communication device are:

- Software compatibility (e.g. Windows, Apple). Some devices come with pre-installed specialist communication software; other software can be purchased as an add-on.

- Portability: size and weight; whether there is a carry handle, strap or stand.

- Access options: All devices considered are touchscreen unless otherwise specified. Multiple-access options means that they can also be accessed with switches and alternative mice like a trackball or joystick. Eye-gaze compatible devices are specified.

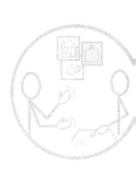

- Mounting: The larger dedicated communication devices tend to come with mounting brackets for wheelchairs, rolling mounts or desk mounts.

- Reliability: processor-size is important when a device needs to run a number of greedy programmes, for example if the user requires eye-gaze or curriculum software alongside their vocabulary software.

- Robustness: children need robust devices, as they will not always position their device carefully. Epilepsy or challenging behaviour may mean the device will be dropped.

- Battery life: most AAC users will want to use their device for most of the day. A solution to extend battery life is hot-swappable batteries.

- Whether this will be a dedicated communication device (often recommended for children, to avoid distractibility) or a multi-function computer (often recommended for young people and adults).

- Aesthetics: this will depend on the user's personal aesthetic preferences. Colourful cases can be an option for children; adults may prefer something more subtle and sophisticated.

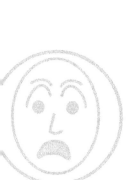

Table 6.8 Name of device

Name of Device	Supplied by:	Software Compatibility (software shown in bold is pre-installed)	Features (Numbers typically related to screen size in inches)
iPad	Various outlets	iOS only	Three screen sizes: iPad mini: 8″ iPad Air 2: 10″ iPad Pro: 10″ and 13″ Lightweight and small tablet. As communication devices, iPads require a robust case, e.g. Griffin Survivor, Kensington. Amplification is also recommended, e.g. Chatwrap (these are not yet available for iPad Pro). May need to use "Guided Access" to lock a child into the communication app, to avoid the child accessing other apps and functions. A good solution for users who do not need other specialist software or access needs and who do not require a rugged device.

Accent	Liberator	**NuVoice** LAMP Unity easyChat Grid 3 (and others: see website)	Three screen sizes: Accent 800: 8″ Accent 1000: 10″ Accent 1400: 14″ (suitable for eye-gaze) Extremely really reliable and robust devices. Long battery life (especially the 1000, with 13–15 hours). Excellent carry handles and stands. Loud speaker. Multiple access options. Keyguards available. Fairly heavy compared with other devices of the same screen-size. Can now be purchased without NuVoice. A good solution for users who have complex access needs.
Chat Fusion	Liberator	LAMP Saltillo	Chat Fusion 8 Chat Fusion 10. Another robust device. Long battery life. Wireless charging on a docking stand. Good carry handle and stand. Relatively lightweight. Multiple access options, including head-pointer. Mounting plate included. A good solution for those requiring specialised access, including head-pointer, but there is no eye-gaze option.

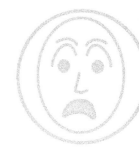

(Continued)

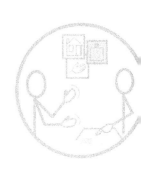

Table 6.8 (Continued)

Name of Device	Supplied by:	Software Compatibility (software shown in bold is pre-installed)	Features (Numbers typically related to screen size in inches)
Liberator Rugged 7 (LR7)	Liberator	**LAMP** **Saltillo**	7″ screen. Extremely robust device with resistance to water, dust and scratches. Direct access only; stylus included. Very long battery life (20+ hours!) Lightweight. Sporty/outdoor attractive case. A good solution for active users who do not have complex access needs.
Grid Pad Go	Smartbox	**Grid 3** Windows 10 Compass Mind Express 4	Two screen sizes: Grid Pad Go 8 Grid Pad Go 10 Relatively lightweight devices, with option to use as multi-function computer. Relatively short battery life (5–6 hours). Multiple access options. A good solution for users who do not have complex access needs.
Grid Pad Pro	Smartbox	**Grid 3** Windows 10 Compass Mind Express 4	Three screen sizes: Grid Pad Pro 11 Grid Pad Pro 13 Grid Pad Pro 18 Relatively short battery life (6 hours) but Grid Pad Pro 13 includes a hot-swappable battery to extend life. GridPad Pro 11 and 13 can be mounted on wheelchair; Grid Pad 18 requires a floorstand. Multiple access options, including eye-gaze. Attractive slim casing. A good

Panasonic Toughpad	Various	Compass Grid 3 Mind Express 4 Windows 8	Toughpad FZ-M1: 7″ Toughpad FZ-G1: 10″ Not a dedicated AAC device, so no loudspeaker, but could be paired with an external Bluetooth speaker. Used widely in industry because of its rugged, durable casing. Dust and water-resistant. Long battery life and hot-swappable battery. A good option for users who do not have complex access needs or require a loud speaker.
Tobii Dynavox T-series	Tobii Dynavox	Compass	Three screen sizes: T-7 T-10 T-15 A robust yet slim and lightweight range of Android AAC devices. Choose a dedicated or standard set-up (the latter allowing access to other applications). The Compass software comes with a companion app for Apple or Windows tablets, allowing you to replicate your package on another device. Loud speaker. Multiple access options. Long battery life (10 hours). Keyguards available. Mountable. A good option for users who do not require a specialised access solution.

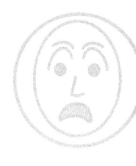

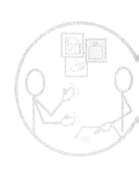

(*Continued*)

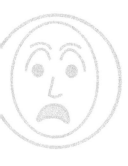

Table 6.8 (Continued)

Name of Device	Supplied by:	Software Compatibility (software shown in bold is pre-installed)	Features (Numbers typically related to screen size in inches)
Tobii Dynavox I-series	Tobii Dynavox	Compass Snap Grid 3 **Mind Express 4** **Windows 10**	Two screen sizes: I-12+ I-15+ Reliable and robust Windows devices. Multi-function computer. Free-standing or mountable. Multiple access options, including built-in Eye-gaze, which gives a very neat device for eye-gaze. "Wake-on-Gaze" feature prolongs battery life. Hot-swappable batteries. Powerful processor: can run multiple AAC programmes, e.g. Grid 3 and Clicker 7 with eye-gaze software. Heavy, but will usually be mounted. A good option for eye-gaze users.
Mobi 2	Techcess	Mind Express 4 Gird 3 **Windows 10**	12" screen. Lightweight and slimline for an eye-gaze device. Multi-function computer. Free-standing or mountable. Multiple access options, including eye-gaze. Integrated mobile phone. Bluetooth module. Extra capacity battery gives 8 hours battery life. A good option for eye-gaze users.

			13" screen.
Tellus 5	Techcess	**Mind Express 4** Compass Grid 3	Reliable and robust. Multi-function computer, including environmental controls. Mountable. Multiple access options, including eye-gaze. Powerful processor: can run multiple AAC programmes, e.g. Grid 3 and Clicker 7 with eye-gaze software. Heavy, but will usually be mounted. A good option for eye-gaze users.
Allora	Techcess	Text-to-speech integrated software	A small dedicated text-to-speech device with an integral keyboard for input (no touchscreen) and small digital text display. Stored phrases and prediction. Recorded message option. An additional mobile display can be given to communication partners to aid their reading of the message. Switch-accessible. Long battery life. SMS texting. Good visibility in bright sunlight. A good solution for cognitively able users who have good language skills, and those with acquired or degenerative conditions.
Lightwriter SL40	Toby Churchill	Text-to-speech integrated software	A small dedicated text-to-speech device with an integral keyboard for input (no touchscreen) and a small digital text display. Stored phrases and predication. Keyguards. Mountable. Environmental controls. Long battery life. SIM card for mobile phone use. Good visibility in bright sunlight. Another good solution for cognitively able users who have good language skills, and those with acquired head injury.

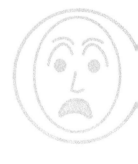

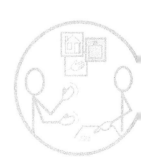

Mainstream devices

Standard PCs, laptops, tablets and even smartphones may be used as AAC devices if they have the processing capability to meet the individual's needs, and if the AAC user does not have specialist access or mounting requirements. The Microsoft Surface Pro and HP Spectre are good examples.

Feature-matching

In the 1990s, Shane and Costello introduced a gold standard of "Feature-Mapping" to help clinicians find the best AAC solution for the client.[17]

The main considerations when choosing an AAC solution are:

- *Symbolic representation*: objects, photos or symbols (WLS/PCS/SymbolStix/ other); single words or pre-programmed phrases. ABC or QWERTY alphabet chart or keyboard.

- *Vocabulary organisation*: Visual Scene Display or Traditional grid layout; Semantic Categories or Pragmatic Functions; predictive grammar; motor-planning or dynamic display.

- *Amount of vocabulary*: a balance of core and fringe vocabulary on every page, or core on a home page and fringe on other pages.

- *Visual acuity and processing*: how much information on each page; colour contrasts; size and layout of cells.

- *Size, weight and portability*: page or screen size; durability of materials; carry handle, strap or stand.

- *Access method*: finger-pointing; fist-pointing; keyguard/touchguide; stylus or dibber; head-pointer; head-mouse; eye-pointing (low-tech), eye-gaze (high-tech), alternative keyboards or mice; trackball, joystick, glidepad; switches (one or two; scanning pattern); eye-pointing (low-tech); eye-gaze (high-tech); partner-assisted scanning.

- *Mounting*: desk mounts/rolling mount/wheelchair mounting.

- *Aesthetics*: the "coolness" factor is also important. This is going to involve personal taste. One AAC user might like a sleek, lightweight design, while another likes a rugged, off-road design. Wireless accessories are often preferred.

Some degree of trial-and-error is inevitable. We have never "finished" with an AAC system. It will always be a work in progress. Additional vocabulary will be needed.

Sentence building and literacy will improve. The communication contexts will evolve. There may be changes in sensory or physical skills. Knowledge of the system will grow. Operational, strategic, social and linguistic competence will improve. New solutions will be needed!

In the next chapter we will look at *alternative access* and *mounting* solutions.

Many types of AAC

Adult AAC users tell us that they also use many different modes of communication, and favour different types of AAC for different situations. There is no AAC hierarchy from no-tech through to low-tech and light-tech and on to high-tech. They are often used concurrently, just as verbal and non-verbal communication modes are used to support one another. Michael Williams,[18] an adult AAC user, says:

> **No one communication mode (an AAC device, a low-tech board, gestures, signs, speech), for example, could possibly meet all my communication needs. I use multiple communication modes – I communicate in many ways. I select the best mode depending on the location, with whom I am communicating and the purpose and content of the communication.**

It is easy to assume that there is a progression from no-tech to low-tech to light-tech to high-tech. However, it is not a hierarchy. We need a balance of each element. Different AAC methods will be used in different situations.

I would like to illustrate this with *the AAC rocket*.

The AAC rocket is built from different components. We need a balance of no-tech, low-tech, light-tech and high-tech. This will be a constantly evolving process: repairs and modifications will need to take place throughout the voyage!

We need a *supportive environment* from the start. This includes home, nursery, school, further education, work and leisure. There needs to be something to talk about, and the opportunity to communicate throughout the day.

We need *Aided Language Stimulation*, provided by responsive conversation partners. This will include strategies to develop attention and listening, play, receptive and expressive language, and literacy skills.

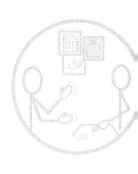

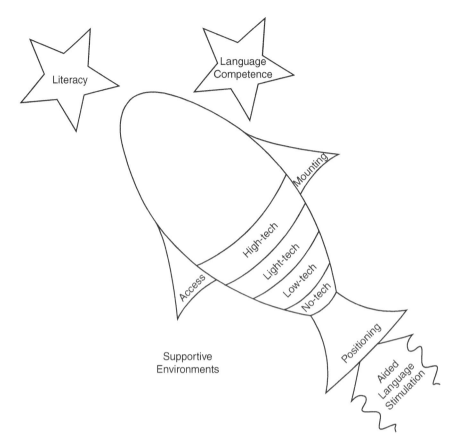

Figure 6.45 AAC rocket

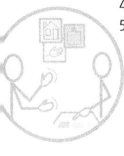

We want our rocket to reach for the stars. The nearest star is *language competence*.[19] *Literacy* will allow exploration of further galaxies.

Notes

1 http://communicationmatters.org.uk. Information on NHS England commissioning is available at http://england.nhs.uk, *Guidance for Commissioning AAC Services and Equipment*, on NHS Education for Scotland at http://nes.scot.nhs.uk, with the excellent resource *IPAACKS: Informing and Profiling Augmentative and Alternative Communication (AAC) Knowledge and Skills*, on NHS Wales at http://whssc.wales.nhs.uk and on services in Northern Ireland on http://online.hscni.net.

2 http://gov.scot/Resource/0039/00394629.pdf.

3 From http://england.nhs.uk, *Guidance for Commissioning AAC Services and Equipment*.

4 http://callscotland.org.uk.

5 See Wilkinson, K., Light, J. and Drager, K. (2012) Considerations for the composition of visual scene displays: potential contributions of information from visual and cognitive sciences. *Augmentative and Alternative Communication*, 28(3), 137–147; see Wilkinson, K. and Light, J. (2011)

Preliminary investigation of visual attention to human figures in photographs: Potential considerations for the design of Aided AAC visual scene displays. *Journal of Speech Language and Hearing Research*, 54(6), 1644–1657.

6 See http://mndassociation.org for more information about voice-banking.

7 http://inclusive.co.uk.

8 http://inclusiveinclusive.co.uk/events/webinars/archive.

9 http://techcess.co.uk.

10 http://callscotland.org.uk/information/text-to-speech/naturalreader/.

11 http://inclusive.co.uk.

12 http://cricksoft.com/uk.

13 http://boardmakeronline.com or http://tobidyanavox.co.uk.

14 http://inclusive.co.uk.

15 http://cricksoft.com/uk.

16 http://penfriend.biz.

17 Shane, H. and Costello, J. (1994) *Augmentative Communication and the Feature Matching Process*. Seminar presented at the American Speech-Language-Hearing Association.

18 Williams, M. (2004) Saying it your way. *Alternatively Speaking*, 7(1), 1–2.

19 The four areas of AAC competence are taken from Light, J. (1989) Towards a definition of communicative competence for individuals using augmentative and alternative communication systems. *Augmentative and Alternative Communication*, 5, 137–144. See Chapters 16 and 17 for more information about AAC competence.

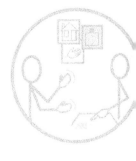

Chapter 7

Alternative access and mounting

Alternative access

Some AAC users will be able to use a touchscreen or a standard keyboard and mouse. Some AAC users will need some modifications. For example, they might need a keyguard on the touchscreen or keyboard, or they might need an alternative mouse, like a joystick or trackball. There will be some AAC users who need further modifications, using a scanning method with switches.

An Occupational Therapist will assess for an AAC user's best access method. This is likely to involve some trial-and-error, and time for the user to learn new skills. One user may use a number of different alternative access methods at different times in the day or for different reasons.

The various access solutions in this chapter may be available to loan through your local AAC Hub, from suppliers, or from local or national AAC organisations. See http://communicationmatters.org.uk for a list of such organisations.

Positioning

Good positioning is of paramount importance. We do not want an AAC user expending unnecessary energy on maintaining their posture, as this will reduce their ability to attend to the communication situation and to operate their communication device.[1]

AAC users who have Cerebral Palsy are likely to need specialist supportive seating to reduce uncontrolled movements and abnormal muscle tone and to inhibit primitive reflexes. An Occupational Therapist and/or Physiotherapist will typically be involved. These professionals will be able to give individual advice, but the general principles of good postural support are:

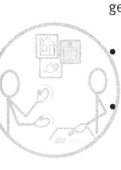

- As symmetrical and upright as is realistic for the individual. Specialist seating may be used.

- The hips, back and shoulders should be stable, possibly using wedges and straps.

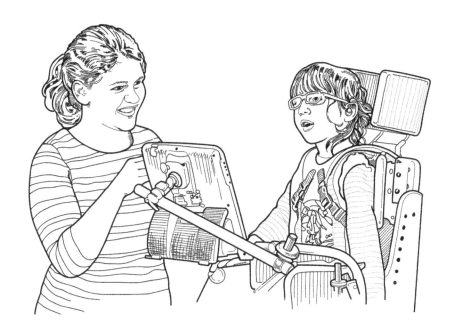

- Seating should be at an appropriate height for hips and knees to be at 90° flexion, with feet flat on the floor or on a footplate.

- A tray may be used to allow elbows to rest comfortably and provide additional postural support and stability.

- The head may be kept in alignment and supported with the aid of a head rest.

- Arms may be supported with a tray or arm rest.

- Position should be changed regularly during the day, so that there are opportunities for standing and reclining.

Direct and indirect selection

Direct selection is where the AAC user can select a desired button or cell without the need for scanning. *Indirect selection* is where switches are used with scanning. Different areas of the screen or individual cells will be highlighted in turn, and the AAC user has to select the one they want. This takes more time and requires more effort.

Direct selection methods include pressing buttons on a keyboard or cells on a touchscreen; selecting a cell with a mouse, trackball, joystick, glide-pad; or using a head-pointer, head-mouse or eye-gaze.

Indirect selection can involve *one switch*, where the device automatically scans the options and the user presses their switch when the desired one is reached; or

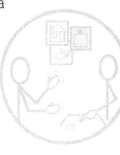

two switches, where the user uses one switch to move the scanner, and the second switch to select. Deciding whether one or two switches are used is dependent on several factors, including managing fatigue and cognitive ability.

Direct selection

Keyboards

A wide range of keyboards is available. There are keyboards with smaller or larger keys. There are keyboards with lowercase or uppercase labels or high-contrast labels on the keys. There are keyboards with colour-coded keys, showing vowels, consonants and numbers in different colours. Keyboard stickers may be added to a keyboard to make the keys more visible for the user. Smaller keyboards are recommended for children, such as the *Cherry Compact* keyboard. One-handed keyboards are also available.

Onscreen keyboards can have a QWERTY, ABC or high-frequency layout. Free onscreen keyboards may not have the necessary clarity, but there are a variety of alternative onscreen keyboards which may be purchased and downloaded as apps. *SuperKeys*[2] is a useful onscreen keyboard for AAC users who have reduced accuracy. When an area of the keyboard is selected, the corresponding cluster of seven keys is enlarged, making selection more accurate.

Keyguards and touchguides

These are covers for touchscreens or keyboards that provide holes for key presses on a keyboard, or cell presses on a touchscreen. They can be made out of metal, perspex or acrylic. A keyguard may be used for an AAC user who would otherwise accidentally press keys or activate cells because of their reduced fine motor control. The keyguard separates the cells and helps to guide their finger, providing tactile feedback too. Touchguides are lighter and thinner than keyguards.

Some manufacturers of communication aids provide keyguards that are compatible with a particular piece of software. In some cases it may be necessary for the AAC Assessment Hub to commission a bespoke keyguard for an AAC device.

Styluses and dibbers

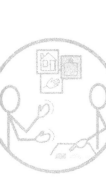

A wide variety of standard and specialist styluses (or dibbers) are available. These might make direct selection less effortful and more accurate. They might have straps or adapted handles that are optimally shaped for the user, and they might be made from an easy-to-grip material. Some touchscreens are capacitive and some are resistive, and the material on the tip of the stylus has to be compatible with the type of touchscreen being used.

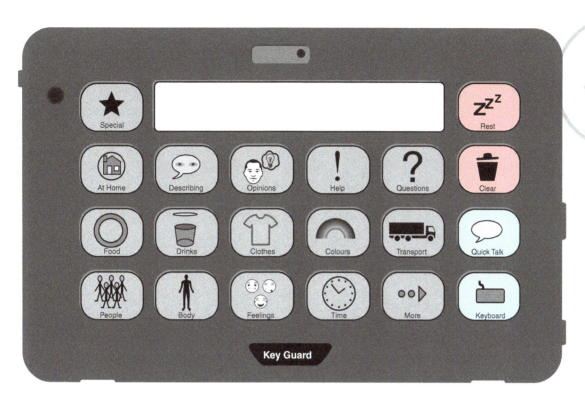

Figure 7.1 Keyguard

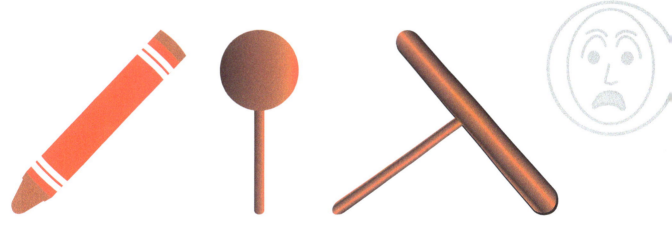

Figure 7.2 Crayon stylus

Figure 7.3 Ball-topped stylus

Figure 7.4 T-bar stylus

Different mice

A range of differently shaped and sized mice are available. Generally, children are more able to use smaller mice. There are also many different designs of ergonomic mice which may be suitable.

Different cursors

Different cursors (pointers) can be downloaded for free from the ACE Centre.[3] These are designed for children with visual processing difficulties who struggle to see a standard cursor on the screen. A wide range of different cursors are available,

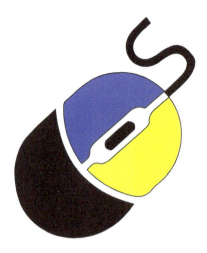

Figure 7.5 Tiny mouse

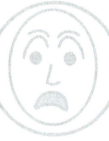

including those that are bigger, more colourful, or animated. The cursor can also be slowed down, or set to leave a trail, in your computer settings. If performing mouse-clicks are problematic, then the cursor can be set to make a selection after a particular *dwell-time*.

Mouse alternatives

Mouse alternatives, like rollerballs and joysticks, tend to be more stable than a conventional mouse, and make it easier to make a selection. Glide-pads tend to be smaller, and may be operated with just a finger or thumb movement, or another part of the body.

Rollerball

These have a large ball in the centre which moves the mouse pointer, and large buttons on either side to allow right- and left-clicks. The whole hand might be used to move the rollerball. Thumb mice, with rollerballs for the thumb, are also available.

Joystick

These have a handle which can rotate to move the screen-pointer, along with various options for performing clicks. There is a range of differently shaped handles.

Glide-pad

These are similar to the glide-pads on a laptop, with different options for clicks. Various sizes and shapes are available. Many can be hand-held and operated by just a thumb or finger, and so can be used by people with a limited range of movement.

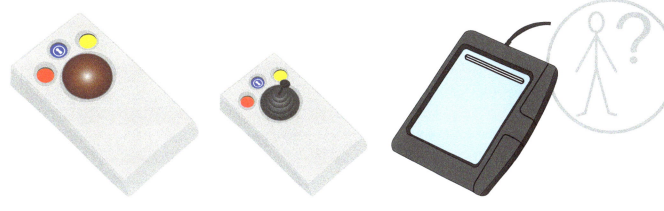

Figure 7.6 Rollerball   **Figure 7.7** Joystick   **Figure 7.8** Glide-pad

Head-pointer

For some AAC users, their head movements may be more accurate than their hand movements. A pointer may be positioned on the head of the AAC user to allow them to control a keyboard or mouse on a computer screen.

Head-mouse

A more subtle head-pointer system comprises a camera on the computer which tracks the head movements of the AAC user, often using a reflective dot placed on the user's forehead or glasses. *Headmouse Nano* and *Tracker Pro*[4] are examples of these devices. *Camera Mouse*[5] is available as a free download for Windows PCs. This head mouse does not require any special equipment, as it uses the webcam in the PC to track head movements. Mouse-clicks can be achieved with dwell-time (fixing on a target for a specified time), or with an alternative mouse or a switch.

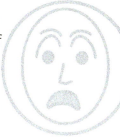

Eye-gaze

Eye-gaze technology is relatively new, and a growth market in AAC. It is important to establish clear terminology when discussing eye-gaze. *Eye-pointing* is a no-tech or low-tech technique, whereby the communicator uses their eyes to point at an object, picture, symbol or letter. *Eye-gaze* is an access method for high-tech AAC or for leisure. A camera, usually placed at the bottom of a computer screen, picks up the movement one or both eyes, and this can then be used to control a pointer on the screen.

Anyone who has ever used eye-gaze will tell you that it is surprisingly effortful to control a pointer on a screen with the eyes. We are used to unconsciously moving our eyes around without thinking about what we are doing. Our eye-movements are very quick and jerky, and without realising, they flick from one place to another. When using eye-gaze, we have to bring this under our conscious control, and very deliberately keep our gaze steady for a set *dwell time* (usually about a

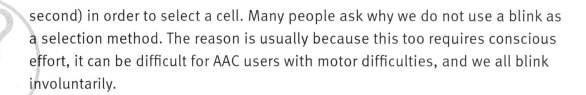

second) in order to select a cell. Many people ask why we do not use a blink as a selection method. The reason is usually because this too requires conscious effort, it can be difficult for AAC users with motor difficulties, and we all blink involuntarily.

New cameras for eye-gaze are being developed all the time. Cameras can pick up both eyes, although they can be set to work with just one eye. Eye colour,[6] glasses,[7] contact lenses[8] and eye conditions,[9] medication, pain and fatigue can all reduce a camera's ability to pick up eye movement, so it is necessary to try equipment to see if it is suitable for the user. An AAC user will need to learn to move their eyes with control and will need to be able to keep a relatively stable head position. The user will also need to dwell on the object and hold their gaze for nearly a second (typically dwell-time is set to 0.9 seconds) to make a selection on a screen. Dwell-free typing is an option for experienced eye-gaze users. Early eye-gaze cameras did not work well in bright sunlight, but again, improvements are being made to cameras.

Eye-gaze for leisure

Most children and adults with profound learning difficulties can access eye-gaze *for leisure*. The camera will pick up their eye-movements and they can passively control the pointer. Some eye-gaze users will continue to use eye-gaze passively, much like in a sensory room, enjoying the light and movement effects.

There are various eye-gaze models being developed, like the *Eye Gaze Software Curve* by CALL Scotland,[10] and handbooks from Inclusive Technology.[11] These detail the component skills needed to progress towards eye-gaze for communication. Complete software packages are available that include a range of games to target these skills, including *Look to Learn*[12] and *HelpKidzLearn EyeGaze*.[13] These do tend to be aimed at younger users, and it is currently a challenge to find age-appropriate activities for older children and adults.

The progression of eye-gaze skills for computer games typically includes:

- *Pre-intentional* gaze. This is essentially passive eye-gaze. The user will accidentally trigger events on the screen. I think of this as being like exploring a sensory room: pre-intentional communicators can enjoy the lights, sounds and movement of sensory stimuli without recognising that they can control what is happening. Fireworks might burst or paint might swirl when the child looks at the screen; the child may or may not realise that they are controlling this.

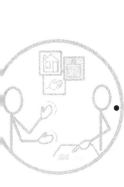

- *Intentional* gaze. This requires an understanding of *cause-and-effect*: I can make something happen just by looking at it! Eye-gaze games like this involve things like popping bubbles and balloons when you look at them. The child might have to work a bit harder, by increasing the "dwell time" before the action occurs.

- *Exploring the whole screen*. An object might pop up in different corners or the top or bottom of the screen. The activities might be similar to those earlier, but with more of a requirement for the child to find the object with their eye-gaze. Alternatively, there may be a visual scene where different actions are triggered by looking at different parts of the screen.

- *Tracking an object*. This may involve tracking a moving object across different areas of the screen, at increasing speeds and with varying patterns. Eye-gaze games may involve following an object to splat it with paint or hit it with a hammer.

- *Making a choice*. This is similar to the "click and select" function with a mouse. It might involve selecting one of two or more objects on the screen to make an action happen. The difficulty level might increase if only one object solves a problem in a sequence of events.

- *Positioning an object*. This is similar to the "click and drag" function on a mouse. It might involve building a picture from stickers or stamps, or completing a jigsaw puzzle. The smaller the object, the more challenging the activity.

Some users will not progress beyond the first stage, but can still use eye-gaze for leisure. Some users will master the latter skills, and show potential for eye-gaze for communication.

Eye-gaze for communication

The skills mentioned previously will help to determine whether an AAC user has the visual skills necessary to progress to eye-gaze for communication. In addition to these though, the child must have certain cognitive, communicative and linguistic skills. These are outlined in the following table.

Visual Skills	
Recognising a picture or symbol on the screen.	This may be assessed in a visual perception test. The user needs to be able to distinguish the image from the background, and recognise it as meaningful, e.g. a flower in a field, rather than pink blobs against a green background. Colour contrasts and size of object and array may be adjusted. OT involvement is essential.

Locating a picture or symbol from an array.	Larger arrays will allow more vocabulary to be used.
Able to move eyes right-left and up-down, separate to head-movement.	For accurate calibration and for using all areas of the screen.
Fixating on one or more areas of the screen.	For moving between different areas or the screen, e.g. from the symbol grid to the sentence bar, and back.
Cognitive Skills	
Understand cause-and-effect.	The child must understand that what they are doing with their eyes is controlling the screen. There is no proprioceptive feedback with eye-gaze, and so it is harder to understand the concept.
Have good memory skills.	The child will need to learn multiple pages of a vocabulary package and efficient navigation pathways.
Social Communication Skills	
Have intentional communication.	The child will need to understand that by looking at a target they can make requests, comments and so on. They may already be doing that by eye-pointing.
Have good attention and listening.	The child will be able to focus for 10–15 minutes in order to practice their eye-gaze skills.
Have a clear yes/no to confirm or repair communication breakdowns.	The child will need to corroborate whether they meant to activate that cell.
Language Skills	
Have symbolic understanding.	The child must show understanding of pictures, symbols or text.
Have receptive language of at least single words.	The child must show understanding of spoken words, e.g. by looking at a named picture.

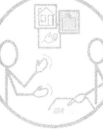

Psychosocial Factors	
Be tolerant of technical problems	This is new technology, so there are likely to be more hardware and software issues.
Is motivated to learn and able to practice.	Eye-gaze for communication requires precise targeting of small areas of screen. The array of cells may need to be reduced at first, with greater spacing between cells. Practice increases proficiency.
Have supportive communication partners.	These partners can support the AAC user in learning eye-gaze skills, and help with trouble-shooting and problem-solving with the AAC Hub.

A much smaller number of children will be able to use eye-gaze as an access method for communication than those who can use it for leisure.

When a person is learning to use eye-gaze, they should take regular breaks, at least every 15 minutes. Practiced users will be able to increase their time. In the early stages, eye-gaze should only be used once or twice per day. Signs of eye fatigue include watery eyes and rapid blinking. It is recommended that another backup access method is also used, for example switching (see later section).

Eventually an AAC user may be able to use a complete symbol-based or text-based vocabulary package, and access curriculum software such as *Clicker*. At first the number of cells on the screen are likely to be limited, with larger target areas. Careful consideration of foreground and background colours is needed. The AAC user can give feedback about adjustments.

The ultimate aim would be to access all computer functions, including web browsers and social media. Menus and links can be accessed through enlarged areas or buttons on the screen. Eye-gaze can also be used for wheelchair-driving and environmental controls.

To summarise, eye-gaze is an exciting development in direct access for high-tech AAC. For a competent eye-gaze user, this can be a quicker and less effortful access method than switching. However eye-gaze for communication takes a lot of practice, and is not a "quick fix". We typically recommend that eye-gaze users develop their eye-gaze skills alongside their switch skills, as they are likely to need both access methods for different purposes, or at different times of the day.

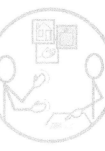

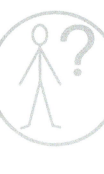

Eye-gaze for assessment

Eye-gaze is usually used as an *output* method, to control what is happening on a screen. An exciting development is also that eye-gaze technology can also be used as an *input* method.[14] New software allows us to see on the screen what a child is looking at, by showing a visual tracker, such as a heat map, as the child looks at different parts of the screen. This can give us an insight into what a child is interested in, their visual skills, and their understanding of spoken language, as they respond to what we say to them. This can be recorded, along with the audio prompts, for analysis.

Indirect access

Switches

Switches are another means of making something happen on a communication device. A wide range of switches are available, which can be activated by almost any part of the body, including the thumb, foot, head, chin and tongue. Switches can be a number of different shapes, including buttons and levers of various sizes. These can be mounted onto wheelchairs at various angles.

For AAC users with very limited movement, electromyographic (EMG) switches can make use of tiny muscle movements, for example in the jaw, brow, or chest. Professor Stephen Hawking uses an infrared switch mounted on his spectacles, and activates this with a cheek muscle twitch.

Switches offer a whole world of opportunity for users with a wide range of physical, sensory and cognitive skills. Feedback from the switch is important: some people like the click or feel of the switch as it is activated. Larger switches require less activation force than smaller switches. For those with multiple profound disabilities, switches are a brilliant way to develop *cause-and-effect*.

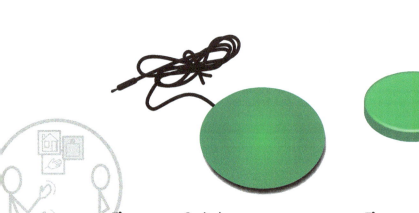

Figure 7.9 Switch

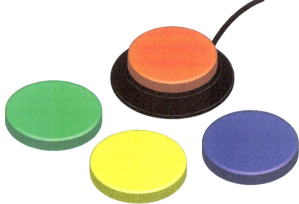

Figure 7.10 Switches

Switch toys and mainstream devices

Whilst specialist switch toys are available, including bubble machines, robots, vehicles and dancing animals, *any* battery or mains-operated device or toy can be switch-operated with the help of a control box such as an *Inclusive Click-On*[15] or an *Ablenet PowerLink*.[16] This means that you can find the right motivator for the user. For example one user might love to turn on music, another might like to turn on a light box.

Switch interfaces

Switches can be wireless (with a Bluetooth connector). Be aware though that the battery drains quickly, and this can lead to user frustration. Switches can be connected to *switch interfaces* for plugging into computers. Switch interfaces can allow the use of multiple switches for different functions. They can be set up to allow for scanning at different speeds, and can be set up for different mouse functions (e.g. click-and-drag).[17] There are now switch interfaces available for tablets.[18]

Switch computer games and apps

There are excellent cause-and-effect computer games available, like the *BigBang*[19] series from Inclusive Technology and *HelpKidzLearn*.[20] These are switch-accessible, but can also be used with mice, rollerballs and joysticks. There are some very good packages of switch games available, including *SwitchIt! Maker*[21] *and ChooseIt! Maker*.[22]

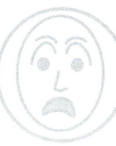

iPad and android tablets can now be made switch-accessible with switch interfaces such as the *APPlicator*[23] and *SimplyWorks*.[24] By using a switch interface for a tablet

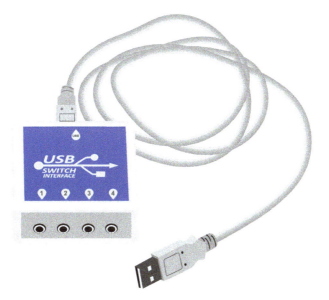

Figure 7.11 Switch interface

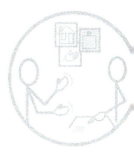

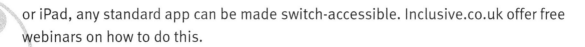

or iPad, any standard app can be made switch-accessible. Inclusive.co.uk offer free webinars on how to do this.

Switches for AAC and computer access

Switches offer a way into high-tech communication aids for cognitively able users. Some users will progress quickly through switch skills. These skills may include using one or two switches (see later) and mouse-functions such as *click-and-hold, click-and-drag*. Ultimately, switches can allow an individual to access all applications on a computer, including an onscreen keyboard.

Inclusive Technology have produced *The Switch Progression Road Map*,[25] which details the stages of switch skills, with ideas for games and activities at each stage. This resource explains how to avoid "switch-banging" (whereby the child repeatedly hits the switch without apparent understanding of cause-and-effect). The resource recommends supervising the AAC user, providing hand-under-hand support if necessary, and varying games and activities to avoid boredom.

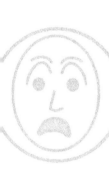

When using switches, it is important for the facilitator to prompt the AAC user correctly. Instead of "hit the switch", give a meaningful prompt like "can you make it work?" or "what could you say?" Ensure that the same consistent command is given at home and in school, to reduce the cognitive load on a child.

One switch or two?

If a user uses one switch, the device will need to be set up to automatically scan through the cells, by row, column or block, before an individual cell is selected. The user will need to learn to wait for the desired area and cell to be scanned before activating their switch. The timing of the scan will need to be personalised. Using one switch requires a lot of cognitive effort to attend to the scanning and to activate the switch on time. Professor Stephen Hawking uses this method of scanning to access an onscreen keyboard.

If a user can use two switches, they can control the scanning with one switch, and select with the other switch. This gives them more control and may be faster. However, it involves more physical effort, involving two parts of the body. Cognitive load is high when learning this pattern, but it is likely to become automatic.

Mounting

We want the AAC user to be using an optimal position, particularly when using a computer-based solution. Mounting ensures that the device and accessories are positioned in consistent positions to minimize the physical effort required to operate the AAC system, and to maximize the user's sensory and motor abilities. The local Spoke Service will be able to provide some mounting solutions. However for clients with very complex needs, where a bespoke solution is necessary, this will come under the remit of the Hub Service.

Wheelchair mounting

Whether a device can be mounted onto a wheelchair will depend on the wheelchair. Lightweight, sporty models may not provide the stability necessary to support a mounted communication aid. In powered wheelchairs, controls for driving and for operating environmental controls and an AAC device may be integrated. However if there is a fault with one system, this impacts on all applications.

It is important for the Hub and Spoke AAC Services to liaise with the Wheelchair Service and the AAC user, to arrive at the best solution for the client.

This is a bespoke solution, and requires trained professionals to correctly fit and adjust the mounting pole, to make any adjustments and carry out stability-testing and risk-assessments.

Rolling floor mount

If an AAC user has a variety of chairs (e.g. a static chair and a wheelchair and a standing or walking frame), then a rolling mount may be the best solution. This is height-adjustable, and can be angled optimally for the AAC user's position. Rolling mounts work well in a client's home so long as there is adequate space for it to be moved around.

Desk mount

For children at school or adults in further education or the workplace, a desk mount is often the best solution. This is a very sturdy frame, which is height-adjustable and can be angled appropriately. A desk-mount, whilst heavy, is a smaller mount than a rolling-mount, and can be moved between classrooms and work-spaces if needed.

Sticky mats

Sticky mats such as *Dycem*[26] mats allow AAC and AT equipment to stay in place on desks and other surfaces. This is especially helpful for AAC users who may have uncontrolled movements, or who cannot easily grade the pressure of their movements.

Mounting for alternative mice and switches

Mats and mounts may be used, which have a sticky, Velcro or suction surface to secure alternative mice and switches. Examples include the *Splatz* switch mount,[27]

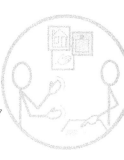

Maxess tray and switch mounts[28] and the *Cling!* plate.[29] Brackets and mounting arms are also available (e.g. *Flexzi*[30] and *Gooseneck*[31] switch mounts). Arm and hand supports with cuffs or straps to support the arm are also available (e.g. *Grip* switch mount).[32]

Mainstream mounts and slopes

A range of standard mounts and writing slopes are available, including *Kensington*[33] mounts and *Posturite*[34] slopes. Low-, light- or high-tech AAC equipment might be placed on these to improve the accuracy of pointing.

Relaxing and reclining

There will be times when a more relaxed position is needed, for example in bed or on the sofa, in the back of a car or on the train. Bean-bag and cushion mounts are available, such as *Trabasack* curve and lap-desk[35] and the *iPad/Tablet Padded Pillow Stand*.[36]

Notes

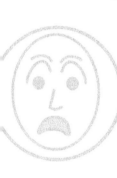

1 Jones, M. and Gray, S. (2005) Assistive technology: Positioning and mobility. In Effgen, S. K. (ed.), *Meeting the Physical Therapy Needs of Children*. Philadelphia, PA: F. A. Davis.
2 This is used in *Crick* software, like *Clicker* programmes, and can be purchased as an app to be used as an alternative iPad onscreen keyboard.
3 http://acecentre.co.uk.
4 http://liberator.co.uk.
5 http://cameramouse.org.
6 Very dark irises are generally harder for an eye-gaze camera to pick up.
7 Lined bifocals can be difficult for the eye-gaze camera to pick up. An anti-reflective coating helps the camera to pick up eye-movements for a user who wears glasses.
8 Contact lenses which move around a lot, or which are weighted to correct astigmatism are more problematic.
9 Cataracts, strabismus, nystagmus, diplopia, hemianopia, dry eye, eye tremor, droopy eye, squint, fluctuating eye dominance, asymmetric pupils, mineral deposits in the eyes or involuntary eye movements can all be problematic.
10 http://callscotland.org.uk.
11 *Inclusive Eye Gaze: Your Essential Guide to Eye Gaze in the Classroom*, free download from http://helpkidzlearn.com, including the *myGaze Learning Wheel*.
12 http://tobidynavox.com and http://smartbox.com.
13 http://helpkidzlearn.com.
14 For example the *Tobii Gaze Viewer* or the *Heat Maps* in Smartbox's *Look to Learn*.
15 http://inclusive.co.uk.
16 http://ablenetinc.com.

17 For example the *Crick USB Switch Box*, or the *Inclusive MultiSwitch 2*, from http://inclusive.co.uk.
18 For example the *APPlicator for iPad* from http://inclusive.co.uk.
19 http://inclusive.co.uk.
20 Ibid.
21 Ibid.
22 Ibid.
23 Ibid.
24 Ibid.
25 Ibid.
26 http://activemobility.co.uk/dycem-slip-mats.
27 http://inclusive.co.uk.
28 Ibid.
29 Inclusive.co.uk
30 http://liberator.co.uk.
31 http://inclusive.co.uk.
32 Ibid.
33 Widely available from various retailers.
34 http://posturerite.co.uk.
35 http://trabasack.com.
36 http://amazon.co.uk.

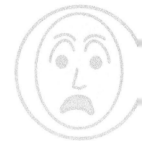

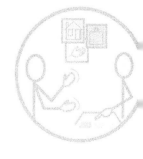

Chapter 8

Why are we afraid of AAC?

AAC might stop the child talking!

This is a common fear, but research shows that introducing an AAC system has a positive effect on speech output. A research review by Millar, Light and Schlosser[1] concluded that of the 27 cases that provided the best evidence, increases in speech production were observed in 89% (24 of 27 cases). In the remaining three cases (11%), there was no change in speech production. None of the 27 cases showed a decrease in speech production as a result of AAC intervention.

In my clinical practice, I cannot tell you how many times a parent or teacher has told me that a child's speech has improved since the introduction of signing or symbol support. VOCAs (Voice Output Communication Aids) provide a highly consistent speech sound model, and this seems to help some children improve their speech sound accuracy. The same child might have undergone blocks of speech sound therapy with no improvement, and then the gains seem almost accidental following the introduction of a VOCA.

Not all children will improve their speech. In the preceding review, 11% didn't. But there may well have been improvements in other aspects of their communication and language-learning. In fact AAC may well kick-start language development.

Attention and listening is likely to improve because adults will tend to use AAC to talk about what the child is interested in. Whilst AAC can be demanding on a child's attention skills, it offers opportunities to practise coordinating looking and listening, and switching attention between an interesting event and the AAC, and back again.

Play and levels of engagement are likely to improve if activities are chosen that are meaningful and accessible for the child, taking into account their sensory, physical, cognitive, language and social communication needs.

Receptive language is likely to improve following the introduction of AAC because language is made more tangible. A sign or symbol can give a clue as to the word's meaning. We can see how a phrase is constructed if we see a symbolised phrase.

Expressive language is likely to improve, because you are giving the child a means to express themselves. They experience the power of communication to request, reject, comment and so on.

No individuals in the study by Millar et al. showed reduced speech after the introduction of AAC. This is worth stressing to parents and carers.

The testimonials or experiences of other parents may be helpful in gaining the support of new parents to AAC. Parent groups for children using AAC are recommended, as a way of offering informal support and information. The NHS[2] have made a video about Toby Hewson, an adult AAC user who is also a company director, talking about what AAC has meant for him. This is also available on the Communication Matters website.[3]

AAC might make the child lazy!

Speech is by far the quickest and easiest way to communicate. No child would choose to communicate using AAC if they had speech available to them. AAC is more effortful, time-consuming and frustrating than speech. If a child is not using speech, but is using AAC, it is not laziness that is stopping them talking. There is a more complicated reason or set of reasons (physical, sensory, cognitive, language or social communication).

We can understand everything that they say

Parents are very good at interpreting their child's non-verbal communication. They are highly attuned to every facial or body movement, however subtle. They can intuitively follow their child's train of thought, because they know their child intimately. They share the same associations and experiences.

But there will come a time when a child's thoughts cannot be guessed. They will be thinking about something unexpected or more complicated than can be conveyed by answering yes or no to skilled questions.

I would like to illustrate this point with help from a young woman called Amy. Amy has four-limb Cerebral Palsy. She has been educated in a special school. At the age of 15, her level of understanding was not known, and she had no means of expression. It was presumed that she was not literate. Amy was assessed by the AAC Hub. The team decided to give Amy access to a text-based communication package. Within a few weeks, Amy wrote the following story:[4]

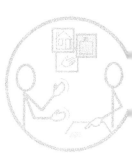

The Party

The night peered in through the window as I got ready for the evening. I was just about ready for the magic to come. I was dressed in a dress as blue as the sky on a summer's jewel like day. The dress had a pattern of white spirals starting at the bottom and going up to the waist which was captivating to the eye. I had sparkly red shoes on like the shoes from the Wizard of Oz. On my cheek I had three small stars shinning in superior silvery glitter. My hair was plaited and fell across my shoulder like a waterfall.

Across the field came the drum beats calling out 'come and join us' 'come and join us'. I obeyed their call drawn like a moth to a flame but hoped I wouldn't get burned tonight. When I arrived the party was not very busy as we were early. However as I looked around I saw the drummers had piled the fire high and it was blazing merrily.

I sat and listened to the fire, which crackled, like the rice crispies I ate for breakfast this morning. It was dancing moving like a ballet dancer performing for the last time and giving it all it had. It was mesmerising.

While I was listening and watching the fire, the drummers picked up the pace and over the hill came some fire jugglers

They juggled around my seat and the field and then when they had finished they put the sticks into the fire. The fire accepted them gratefully and killed them with a bang.

Marshmallows appeared and were roasted and I was given one. It tasted of liquid gold, still warm from the fire.

At the break of dawn I went to bed tired but happy.

—Amy Clark

No one would have been able to guess that these ideas were inside Amy, or that she would be able to use language to such beautiful effect.

AAC is different!

Most people have had very limited exposure to AAC. There are misconceptions about AAC. Most people will confuse Makaton with British Sign Language. They will confuse signs with symbols. They will recognise Stephen Hawking, but have no idea how he talks. You can explain what AAC stands for, but then you have to explain what Augmentative and Alternative Communication means. It is very difficult for people to get the idea just by hearing the words. I think you have to see AAC in action to actually get it.

Once you see what an AAC user can do with AAC, you understand how important it is, and then it doesn't matter so much that it is different. And it isn't *that* different. We all use gestures, which are similar to signs. We all use icons on our desktop and phone, which are similar to symbols. We do need to be sensitive to AAC users' concerns that they do not want to look too different. AAC devices now look and sound more mainstream than they did 10 years ago: the devices tend to be more attractive, and the software incorporates elements of mainstream software, such as synthesised speech and social media compatibility.

AAC is complicated!

You have to learn various skills in order to use AAC. It *is* complicated. But you should be able to access support. Start with one AAC user, with one type of AAC, and take it step by step. Learn the best way to cue or prompt this AAC user. Learn how to read their "yes" and "no". Watch someone else who knows the AAC user well, and copy what they do. Like any new skill, or set of skills, at first this will seem really hard and effortful. You will have to concentrate, and you will make lots of mistakes. That is normal, just like riding a bike, swimming or driving. Eventually, it will start to come more easily, and you will build a set of skills to help this AAC user. You will find that many of these skills are just as useful for other AAC users. You will be interested to find that there are huge individual differences between AAC users and their AAC systems, and that this is really interesting. AAC is fascinating because it is complicated!

Technology is intimidating!

Depending on the generation that you belong to, technology may or may not be intimidating. If you were born after 1985, then you probably won't read this section. If you were born before 1985, you probably remember some degree of confusion or even incomprehension when you first heard about computing, the internet, emailing, or Twitter. You may remember setting up a PC or smartphone for the first time, and being intimidated. Like all new skills, it is hard at first, but it gets easier.

If you need a hand to hold, then ask for support. Get someone else to show you. A few times. Don't be frightened of asking stupid questions, because that is how you learn.

Learn as you go along, on a "need to know" basis. If you are a parent or a teacher of a child getting their first AAC device, then just get used to using the device before you learn how to program it.

If your child, or a child you are working with, is using a symbol-based package, it's a good idea to spend some time on your own becoming familiar with where the different symbols are located so that you feel more confident to use the VOCA in everyday communication. Try to do this in a practical way by thinking how you would use the device to say something specific, for example, what you did at the weekend and how you felt about it. There will inevitably be symbols you cannot find. Try to find ways around this: if you can't find "ostrich", then say "big bird". When you can't find a symbol when you are with the child, then talk through your thought processes as you try to find it: for example, "it's something we eat, so I'll look in 'food and drink' ". It's OK to make mistakes: AAC users need to see that it is OK to have a go and risk failure – even better if we can model repairing a mistake.

If you are a Speech and Language Therapist, use your CPD time to have a go at making a low-tech support, like a "now and next" board. There should be someone in your department who can show you, and if there isn't, then flag this up with your manager. Every Speech and Language Therapist should have access to some form of symbol software: it is as essential to the role as a mirror!

Software providers and AAC Hubs offer training, including webinars. User guides are provided with the software, or you can email or ring the company with queries.

The Specialist AAC companies are responsive to customer feedback. They are constantly working to improve the "user interface" of their products.

Technology goes wrong!

Yes, it does. The newer the technology, the more likely it is to go wrong. Therefore, no-tech, low-tech and light-tech AAC are an essential balance to high-tech. If a high-tech device needs to go in for repair for a few days, then the AAC user needs to have a backup means of communicating.

Tolerance of technical glitches is individual. It is one of the factors that a Hub Assessment will consider for an individual. The Hub should explain pros and cons of various high-tech solutions, including how reliable a device or software package is. Hubs can respond very quickly to technology issues, as many are easily fixed. There will be occasional breakages which will require the device to be sent back to the manufacturer. Hub services generally have a like-for-like loan device available, or the manufacturer can supply one if the device is under a warranty or aftercare package.[5] Some of the most exciting technology is the most unstable, but this may be tolerated by a user who benefits from the technology and who has backup AAC.

The array of AAC choices is overwhelming . . .

There is a natural tendency for professionals to develop "favourite" AAC solutions, because they become familiar with these. It is important that every potential AAC user is seen as an individual. They have a unique profile of physical, sensory, cognitive, linguistic and communication abilities, communication environments and personal preferences. We must include the AAC user and their family in our decision-making to find the best fit for the individual.

AAC professionals need to keep up to date with developments in the field by reading research, attending workshops, training or conferences. They need to be in touch with AAC users through online forums and newsletters. The AAC field is relatively small, and so it is not hard to be part of the community. Communication Matters is the UK AAC charity, and offers a wealth of information and resources for AAC professionals.[6]

AAC is expensive for schools!

If a child or young person is in an educational provision, then they should have access to aids and equipment that enable their participation under the Equality Act 2010.[7] All schools are provided with funding to meet the needs of children and young people with Special Educational Needs and Disabilities. Schools are able to apply for additional top-up funding if the resources needed to support a child exceed the nationally prescribed threshold per pupil per year. Funding for a bespoke high-tech AAC device for an individual comes from Regional or National AAC Hubs and not the school. However the school is expected to provide more mainstream AAC resources such as curriculum software and access to a suitable computer.

Therapy resources are limited!

There is now a network of Regional and National Specialised AAC Assessment Centres across the UK.[8] This has been developed to ensure equality of access to services. In England this service provision is known as the "Hub and Spoke" model. Scotland, Wales and Northern Ireland operate equivalent models. Local, or Spoke Services are commissioned to work with Regional, or Hub Specialised AAC Assessment Centres. Where there is a skills gap in the Local Spoke service, the Regional Hub Service can support with training. Hub and Spoke loan banks of equipment are available for trials of equipment.

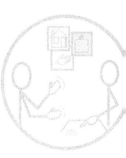

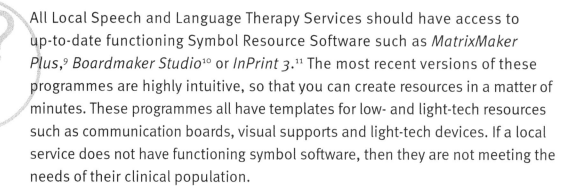

All Local Speech and Language Therapy Services should have access to up-to-date functioning Symbol Resource Software such as *MatrixMaker Plus*,[9] *Boardmaker Studio*[10] or *InPrint 3*.[11] The most recent versions of these programmes are highly intuitive, so that you can create resources in a matter of minutes. These programmes all have templates for low- and light-tech resources such as communication boards, visual supports and light-tech devices. If a local service does not have functioning symbol software, then they are not meeting the needs of their clinical population.

Time is limited!

Creating AAC resources is an essential element of a care package for an individual with identified need. Interventions are a balance of direct therapy time and indirect intervention, including the preparation of resources. It is fantastic if there is a Therapy Assistant or Teaching Assistant to help with the creation of these resources. I would recommend that Therapists and Teachers create at least some resources so that they have knowledge of the process, and can give adequate guidance to the assistant. This is a creative process which is highly rewarding. You are giving a child a voice!

We need training!

Yes, you do. This is an essential element of a child's AAC intervention. Regional AAC Hubs provide training for Local Spoke Services. Some training then may be offered by the Spoke Service to parents, schools and partner agencies. These arrangements will be locally agreed, with Hub and Spoke Services working together to determine the levels of expertise in the Spoke Service. The more bespoke the solution for an individual, the more likely it is that the Hub Service will provide some level of training or mentoring for the AAC user and their family and partner agencies, and Local Spoke Services.

We need support!

Yes, you do. This is what Regional Hubs are for. Support may take the form of face-to-face training and mentoring, remote webinars, conference calls, emails or phone calls. Planning meetings, consultations, Education, Health and Care Plans (EHCP) and transition meetings are all forums when support needs can be identified and an action plan put into place. Hub and Spoke Services will work together to provide an assessment and intervention plan that is individualised for the child, family and services supporting them.

It is essential that professionals identify where they need support. It is not expected that every Speech and Language Therapist, Occupational Therapist or Specialist Teacher will know everything there is to know about every AAC solution. That would be impossible. It is important to know what you don't know, rather than feeling pressure to fake expertise! AAC users and their families appreciate honesty and a willingness to learn.

We've tried this before and it didn't work!

There may be history here. The potential AAC user and their family may have experienced a sense of failure with AAC before. Acknowledging any fear or scepticism is an important step in enabling people to move on and risk failure again. The team around the child may be able to identify why they feel the time is right now, and what support needs to be in place.

As professionals we need to judge whether an individual is ready for an AAC solution. Because of the wide range of AAC solutions, there aren't really any individuals who aren't ready for AAC due to their cognitive level.[12] It may not feel like the right time for their family, but this is an ethical issue we need to carefully consider. We need to provide individuals and their families with appropriate information so that they can make an informed decision.

For young people aged over 16, we should assess mental capacity.[13] This can be combined with using opinion charts or *Talking Mats*[14] for advocating the person's views about their communication and AAC. There are basic communication standards that vulnerable adults can expect from residential settings.[15] Safeguarding procedures can be implemented if basic standards of care are not being met.

How do I combine AAC with other interventions?

We may need to work on the foundation skills for communication, for example joint-engagement with Intensive Interaction.[16] We may want to give caregivers the interaction skills to promote communication and language development, for example with Parent-Child Interaction Therapy or *Hanen*.[17] We may need to help the family come to terms with a diagnosis, for example of Autism Spectrum Condition.[18] We may need to work on a child's receptive language. We may continue to work on speech sounds. AAC may (and should) be introduced in conjunction with other interventions.

We don't know where to start!

It is important that an AAC intervention is appropriate to the individual. We need to carry out a high-quality assessment of this child's physical, sensory, cognitive and

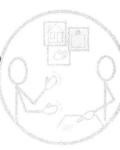

communication needs as part of a multi-disciplinary intervention team. Assessment will initially be carried out by the Local Spoke Service. It could lead to a referral to the Regional Specialised AAC Assessment Hub Service.[19] Hubs offer one-off consultations as well as full assessments, and can also offer advice pre-referral.

Assessment will be covered in Chapter 10. Feature-matching (see Chapter 10) is a useful tool in reaching the right high-tech AAC solution for this individual. It is important that provision of an AAC solution is just the starting point.[20] There needs to be a process of support and training from there. The process is never complete: tweaks and changes are inevitable, and the AAC solution is an ever-evolving process.

I don't know how to move this AAC user on!

We need to work towards four communication competencies identified by Janice Light:[21] Operational, Linguistic, Social and Strategic competency. If an individual is not making progress, there may be psychosocial reasons, like motivation or confidence. There may be barriers in the social environments of the AAC user, like a need for knowledge and training for the staff group. If you are really stuck, contact your Regional AAC Hub for advice or a one-off consultation. Target-setting and EHCPs will be looked at in more detail in Chapter 14.

Notes

1 Millar, D., Light, J. and Schlosser, R. (2006) The impact of augmentative and alternative communication intervention on the speech production of individuals with developmental disabilities: A research review. *Journal of Speech, Language, and Hearing Research*, 49, 248–264.
2 http://nhs.uk/Video/Pages/aac.aspx.
3 http://communicationmatters.org.uk/news-item/2016-aac-video-of-our-co-chair.
4 The spelling and punctuation has been left unedited to show Amy's skills.
5 For example *Libcare* for Liberator devices: see http://liberator.co.uk.
6 http://communicationmatters.org.
7 http://legislation.gov.uk.
8 See Chapter 5 for a fuller description of this model.
9 http://inclusive.co.uk.
10 http://inclusive.co.uk or http://toby-churchill.com.
11 https://widgit.com.
12 Romski, M. (2005) Augmentative communication and early intervention: Myths and realities. *Infants and Young Children*, 18(5), 174–185.
13 www.gov.uk. *Mental Capacity Act Code of Practice*, updated 12 January 2016.
14 http://talkingmats.com.

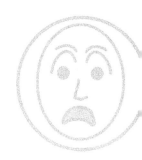

15 http://rcslt.org. *Five Good Communication Standards: Reasonable Adjustments to Communication That Individuals With Learning Disability and/or Autism Should Expect in Specialist Hospital and Residential Settings.*

16 http://intensiveinteraction.co.uk.

17 See http://hanen.org for interventions including *It Takes Two to Talk* and *More Than Words*.

18 For example *EarlyBird*. See http://autism.org.uk.

19 See Chapters 6 and 10 for the referral criteria to a Specialised AAC Assessment Hub.

20 Light, J. and McNaughton, D. (2013) Putting people first: Re-thinking the role of technology in augmentative and alternative communication intervention. *Augmentative and Alternative Communication*, 29(4), 299–309.

21 Light, J. (1989) Toward a definition of communicative competence for individuals using augmentative and alternative communication systems. *Augmentative and Alternative Communication*, 5, 137–144.

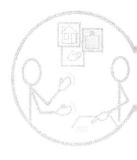

Chapter 9

Aided Language Stimulation

A key message throughout this book is that the child who requires AAC is not that different from any other child. As parents, Teachers and Speech and Language Therapists, we can apply what we already know to working with these children.

I would like to briefly re-visit the *Language Development Pyramid*.

Typically developing children tend to acquire language regardless of the quality of language modelling. There may be differences in vocabulary size,[1] sentence complexity and social use of language[2] depending on the language modelling provided, but even with very limited support, children achieve competency.

Children learning to use AAC need more input from those around them to achieve success. It is not enough to put an AAC resource in front of a child and expect them to start using it.

I have added Aided Language Stimulation to the Language Development Pyramid (see Diagram 9.1). It is represented as the sun because Aided Language Stimulation illuminates language- and AAC-learning for the child.

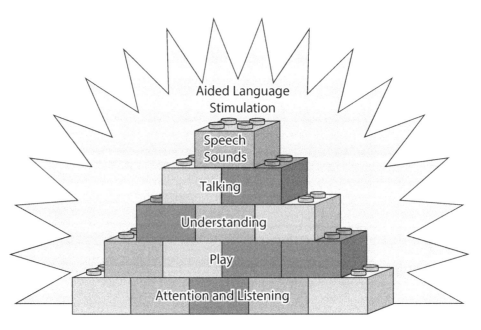

Diagram 9.1 Pyramid and sun (following model of pyramid in Chapter 2)

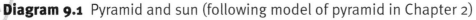

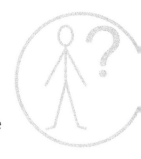

Aided Language Stimulation provides a social context for communication. Children thrive in a social environment where they are seen as delightful and fascinating. The adult is responsive to everything that the child does, and assumes intentional communication. The adult recognises where the child is at now, and provides scaffolding towards the next stage in language development.

Helping children to learn language

We have already seen how caregivers naturally adopt "Parentese" when talking to small children. There are many strategies adults adopt to help children to learn spoken language.[3] These include:

- Being face-to-face to help the child to attend to what we say

- Following the child's focus of interest, and talking about this[4]

- Showing the child what we are talking about

- Using an interesting voice and animated face

- Emphasising and repeating key words

- Simplifying our language to be one step ahead of the child

- Adding one or two words to what the child has said

- Waiting for a response before giving more information

- Responding to everything a child does and interpreting it as meaningful

- Valuing the child's contribution to the interaction

- Using self-talk (talking about what we are doing) and parallel-talk (talking about what the child is doing) throughout the day

- Using a rich and varied vocabulary once the child has learnt the basics

- Expanding upon what the child has said and using more complex sentences

- Encouraging an interest in the sound of language.

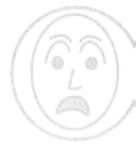

Many speech and language therapy interventions incorporate these natural processes. For example *Parent-Child Interaction Therapy*,[5] *Hanen*,[6] *Intensive Interaction*[7] and *Non-directive Therapy*[8] are largely based on the assumption that the adult can "scaffold" a child's communication and language development, to be one step ahead, thus providing the ideal modelling.

We can do the same with AAC!

Aided Language Stimulation

In typical language development, a child is immersed in a language-rich environment from birth. The child hears spoken language from the moment they wake up to the moment they are tucked into bed at night. We naturally accompany their every movement and thought with a spoken word or phrase. They are exposed to a rich a varied vocabulary, myriad phrases and sentence constructions, and an appropriate range of pragmatic functions in different social situations. We encourage children to babble and play with sounds, words and phrases. These children are learning from experts, because as adults we are competent in spoken language.

We do this because we assume they will learn to speak.

Where a child may not develop spoken language, we may do exactly the right thing and introduce AAC early. We present them with a communication board or book and wait for them to use it.

We might even use it a little bit. Say 10% of our total interaction with them?

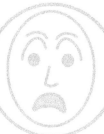

However, if we want them to use signs or symbols expressively, we need to model it receptively. We need to put in before we can get out!

AAC users also need to be immersed in Aided Language Stimulation from the moment they wake up to when they are tucked into bed at night. They do not have the luxury of learning from competent AAC users, so they will have to learn alongside us, as we learn to become competent.

AAC Specialist Jane Korsten[9] has calculated that the average 18-month-old child has been exposed to 4,380 hours of oral language at a rate of 8 hours per day from birth. A child who has an AAC system and receives speech and language therapy two times per week for 20–30 minutes sessions will reach this same amount of language exposure in 84 years. It is therefore vital that AAC Specialists work with parents, carers and teaching staff so that they are able to provide Aided Language Stimulation throughout the day. AAC should be threaded through every daily activity, just as spoken language occurs in every daily activity.

Below are 10 top tips for Aided Language Stimulation. These might be shared with parents, carers and teaching staff.

For a more formal approach, they might be used in Adult- or Parent-Child Interaction Therapy. It is important that such approaches always emphasise

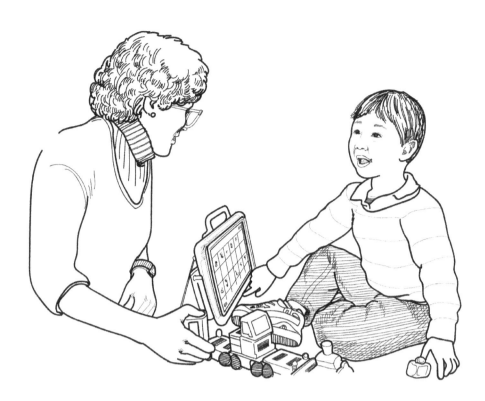

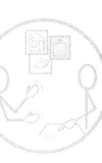

what the communication partner is already doing to support communication. This process should be a positive experience, whereby the communication partner feels valued and their skills are recognised. The communication partner will be comfortable to experiment with making slight adjustments to their communication style when they feel valued. Video can be a useful tool in analysing what the communication partner is doing to support the AAC user.[10] I would recommend that AAC practitioners use video as a self-reflection tool to recognise their own good practice. People are very quick to criticise themselves on video, and it is a skill to focus on the positives, and to build on these.

No communication partner will master the list of skills shown below. Like AAC, this is a constant work in progress!

Ten top tips for Aided Language Stimulation[11]

1 *Be face-to-face.*

Try to make it easy for the child to glance at you regularly whilst they are playing. This will build joint attention, which is vital for language learning. Make sure that the child can also easily see any signs or symbols you will use. Parents of deaf children often sign on their children's faces or bodies, and this has been shown to help the children attend to the sign.[12] We can try to apply this to AAC too. In the very early stages, try to take your sign or your symbol to the child, so that they don't have to put in any effort to look at it. You won't

need to do this forever: once your child is in the good habit of attending to what you are saying, they will naturally shift their gaze from what they are doing to the sign or symbol you use.

2 *Follow what your child is interested in, and talk about this.*

Children are more likely to attend to language when we talk about what they are doing and what they are already interested in. We need to join them in their world, rather than expecting them to join us in our world, because we are the competent communicators. They are just learning. Try to say what you think your child would say, if they could, using their AAC system. If this sounds like a lot to coordinate, that's because it is, and it takes practice. Using your child's AAC system *will* slow you down, and to some extent, that is the point. Slowing down and simplifying what you say will help your child's understanding of language. If your child has good understanding of spoken language, then continue to use full sentences whilst you point out the relevant symbols. You will get a sense of whether your child needs you to simplify your symbolised sentences, or whether they can cope with longer, grammatical sentences. What they say back to you will be a good indication of this.

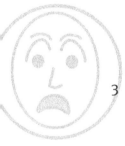

3 *Showing your child what you are talking about.*

At the early stages of language-learning, this may mean holding the object up to the child, or pointing at it, and using a single word, along with a sign or symbol, to label that object. Similarly, if you are labelling an action, you can say the word (e.g. "eat") accompanied by a sign or symbol, then carry out the action. Then you can repeat the word with the sign or symbol, to reinforce it. As your child starts to learn language, you can highlight the *new word* in a phrase. For example if you know that they know the word "bird" and you see a bird flying, you might say "look, bird's *flying*", emphasising the word "flying" as you sign it or show the symbol. You might just repeat this new word with the sign or symbol. Later on, you might be teaching the concept of "dirty". This time you will show the child the dirty socks and you will say "uh, this sock is *dirty*" as you sign or show a symbol for "dirty". You might rephrase this and say "it's a *dirty* sock", again signing or showing a symbol for "dirty". Your face and voice will also convey that "dirty" is not good: you are showing what you mean using every available mode of communication. Try to always teach new language concepts through real-life, multi-sensory experience. This makes language more memorable and meaningful.

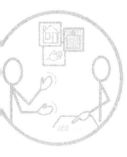

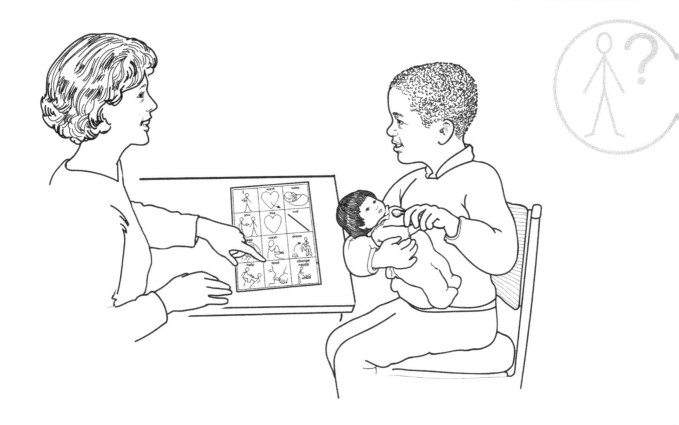

4 *Talk about everything that happens, throughout the day.*

We want our child to have a fully immersive experience of spoken and aided language. Therefore we need to talk about everything, throughout the day, using their AAC system. This may mean we need different AAC modes at different times of the day. For example we might use no-tech signing in the middle of the night. We might use a low-tech communication chart that is laminated and stuck to the bathroom tiles at bath-time. We might have a light-tech single message device near the toilet to say "help me!" or a multi-step device to say what equipment we need to take to school. We might have a high-tech device to chat over breakfast, to engage in learning activities at school, and to play with a sibling at home. This will not come naturally to caregivers: they will have to work at getting to know what the AAC system can and can't do, where vocabulary is stored, and how words or symbols can be combined. Practice will make (almost) perfect.

5 *Respond to, and expand upon everything your child does.*

Assume that your child is being communicative, even if you are not sure. Be sensitive to their mood, and be an empathic communicator. Mirror their body

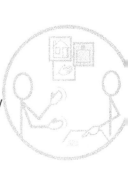

language, facial expression and tone of voice as you interpret their message. There may be times when your child "babbles" with sounds, signs or symbols. Copy back what you think they might have said. You can use a questioning tone of voice to indicate that you're not sure. This might involve you saying and pointing to a different symbol, if you think they meant to say that. If you don't think you got the message, then you can try again, suggesting a different sign or symbol. There may be times when your child talks nonsense using their AAC. This is very normal! You can join in the fun by choosing equally fun symbols, or combining them to make silly phrases (e.g. "you monkey", "daddy gorilla").

6 *Repeat! Repeat! Repeat!*

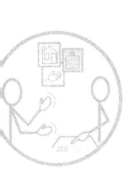

A child learning spoken language takes 5 years to achieve language competence, so they are likely to need at least as long to achieve AAC competence. A child has to hear a word many times before they fully understand its meaning and can use it correctly. If a child has sensory, motor, language or learning difficulties, they may need even more exposures to the word in meaningful everyday situations. Keep plugging away, saying the same words whilst signing them or pointing to the symbol. Don't be disheartened if your child doesn't use the word, sign or symbol straight away. You can experiment with new ways to make the word meaningful for your child. Try to use all of their senses and embed the word in their daily experiences. Once your child has learnt a word, use it in new phrases to build their awareness of syntax and grammar. For example, if they have learnt "ball", then model "ball gone", "more ball", "here ball", "throw ball", "catch ball", "roll ball", "kick ball", "mummy's ball", "Imi's ball", and so on.

7 *Add to what your child says or does.*

If your child is non-verbal, then use single words, accompanied by a sign or symbol. If they use single words, signs or symbols, then repeat back what they said and add a word, to make a two-word phrase. Use their AAC system as you model this two-symbol phrase! If they have good understanding, then you might say a full sentence whilst modelling the two key symbols. For example if your child points to the symbol "hot", you might say "your dinner is hot" as you point to the symbols "dinner" and "hot". You are then modelling spoken language at an appropriate level for their good receptive language, and you are modelling AAC at an appropriate level for their emerging expressive language.

8 *Give your child time to respond.*

Children need four times as long as adults to process language. Add sensory, motor, language or learning difficulties to this, and you may need to allow more processing time. AAC demands more processing time, as the child has to shift their attention from what they are doing, to looking at a sign or symbol. This requires more conscious effort than just listening to a word. You will gradually instinctively know how much time you need to leave before expecting a response from your child, but at first leave longer than you think you need to. Your child's turn might be subtle: it might be a glance, a facial expression or a body movement. You might cue them by moving their AAC system closer, by pointing to it, or by signing to look at it. Try not to overload them with a verbal prompt unless you have waited a sufficient amount of time.

9 *Comment, don't question.*

Children tend to say more when an adult makes a comment, rather than asks a question. For example, if the adult says "you've found a fish", rather than "what have you found?" Asking a question puts the child under pressure, and we all go silent if there is pressure to talk. Commenting provides a model for the child: they get the right word, sign or symbol for the thing they have found or done, so that they can start to understand and use that word if they want to. If you catch yourself asking a question, then answer it for the child (e.g. "what are you doing? You're building!"). When your child is confident with starting conversations, then you can start to ask questions. *What, who and where* questions are more concrete and easier to answer than *when, why and how* questions.

10 *Model how to use the AAC system.*

Show that you value your child's AAC by using it as much as possible. Talk through your thought processes as you try to find a symbol. For example, "I'm looking for *helicopter* . . . I'll look in *transport*." If you can't find a symbol, model using a similar one (e.g. "it's a bit like an *aeroplane*"). The strategies will vary: you may be able to sign the word, to find it on another AAC resource, or you may be able to spell a word out on an alphabet chart. Remind others to use your child's AAC too. Siblings can be fantastic for modelling. Give everyone including your child the message that AAC is a valued method of communication at home, in nursery, school or college,

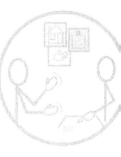

when out and about and so on. Protest if someone "forgets" the AAC, by saying "Oh no! How are you going to communicate if you don't have your chart/book/talker?"

Notes

1   Hart, B. and Risley, T. R. (1995) *Meaningful Differences in the Everyday Experience of Young American Children*. Baltimore, MD: Brookes.

2   Hart, B. and Risley, T. R. (1999) *The Social World of Children Learning to Talk*. Baltimore, MD: Brookes.

3   For example, *Tips for Talking* on http://talkingpoint.co.uk, *Talk Together* on http://icancharity.org.uk and *Listen up* on http://thecommunciationtrust.org.uk; Kaiser, A., Hemmeter, L. and Hester, P. (1997) The facilitative effects of input on children's language development: Contributions from studies of enhanced milieu teaching. In Adamson, L. and Romski, M. (eds.), *Communication and Language Acquisition: Discoveries From Atypical Development*. Baltimore: Paul H. Brookes; Yoder, P., Warren, S., McCathren, R. and Leew, S. (1998) Does adult responsivity to child behaviour facilitate communication development? In Warren, S. and Reichle, J. (Series eds.) and Wetherby, A, Warren, S. and Reichle, J. (Vol. eds.), *Communication and Language Intervention Series Vol. 7. Transitions in Prelinguistic Communication*. Baltimore: Paul H. Brookes, pp. 39–58.

4   Tomasello, M. and Farrar, M. (1986) Joint attention and early language. *Child Development*, 57(6), 1454–1463.

5   Kelman, E. and Schneider, P. (1994) Parent-child interaction: An alternative approach to the management of children's language difficulties. *Child Language Teaching and Therapy*; Falkus, G., Tilley, C., Thomas, C., Hockey, H.,, Kennedy, A., Arnold, T., . . . Pring, T. (2015) Assessing the effectiveness of parent-child interaction therapy with language-delayed children: A clinical investigation. *Child Language Teaching and Therapy*.

6   Girolametto, L. and Weitzman, E. (2006) It takes two to talk – The Hanen Program for parents: Early language intervention through caregiver training. In McCauley, R. and Fey, M. (eds.), *Treatment of Language Disorders in Children*. New York: Brookes, pp. 77–103.

7   Hewett, D. (2011) *Intensive Interaction: Theoretical Perspectives*. London: Sage.

8   Cogher, L. (1999) The use of non-directive play in speech and language therapy. *Child Language Teaching and Therapy*.

9   See http://everymovecounts.net/theauthors.

10 Cummins, K. and Hulme, S. (1997, Autumn) Video: A reflective tool. *Speech and Language Therapy in Practice*, 4–7.

11 If these 10 top tips look remarkably similar to Parent-Child Interaction Therapy, that's because they are! I have just adapted them for use with AAC.

12 See Morgan, G. and Woll, B. (eds.) (2002) *Directions in Sign Language Acquisition*. Amsterdam: John Benjamins.

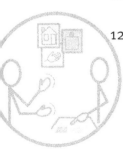

Chapter 10

AAC assessment

In the first instance, a potential AAC user will be referred to the local Speech and Language Therapy service. This may be through Early Support for very young children. Speech and Language Therapy Services have an open referral system, meaning that anyone can refer: the referral does not have to come from a GP or other health professional. Teachers and parents can also refer a child to Speech and Language Therapy.

See the website of the Royal College of Speech and Language Therapists (RCSLT; http://rcslt.org) *How to find an SLT* for up-to-date information about your local Speech and Language Therapy Service.

Hub and Spoke Model of AAC services

The Hub and Spoke Model was introduced in 2014 in England to describe how Local (Spoke) services are to work with Regional (Hub) AAC services. Scotland, Wales and Northern Ireland have equivalent service delivery models for Local and Regional (or National) Specialised AAC Assessment Centres.

The Local or *Spoke Service* is the local team of Speech and Language Therapists, Occupational Therapists and possibly teachers, to whom a child, young person or adult will be initially referred when in need of AAC. They will assess the individual's communication, language, learning, physical and sensory needs, as well as the need for AAC, and will provide no-tech, low-tech and light-tech solutions. They may also provide high-tech solutions if these are fairly mainstream and readily available, for example, communication apps. The Spoke Team will also provide access and mounting solutions and environmental controls if the best solution is fairly mainstream and readily available. For more bespoke solutions to high-tech AAC and environmental control, a referral to the Hub Service will be needed.

For a current list of local Specialised AAC Assessment Hubs, see http://communicationmatters.org.uk. The Hub Service comprises Speech and Language Therapists, Occupational Therapists, and possibly Specialist Teachers and Clinical Scientists or Technicians who have specialist knowledge of high-tech AAC. This team of professionals will work together to provide the best bespoke solution for an individual.

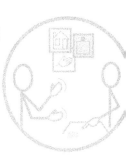

AAC assessment by the local spoke service

This may be from a Speech and Language Therapist alone, or there may be a Multi-disciplinary Assessment. If there is a recognised need for AAC, and the child has multiple impairments (e.g. Global Developmental Delay or additional sensory or motor impairments), the assessment should include an Occupational Therapist. The child or adult may already have had some experience of using AAC. If so, their use and competency should be included in the assessment. A very detailed and comprehensive assessment tool is the *Functional Communication Profile–Revised*.[1] This may be used in its entirety, or relevant sections can be used.

Most formal Speech and Language assessments are not suitable for AAC users because they are only standardised for children or adults who do not have sensory, physical, cognitive or social communication impairments. There are also access issues with a paper-based assessment. However, parts of formal assessments may be used in an informal way, and informal assessments may be used. Assessments which may be useful include the Derbyshire Language Assessment Rapid Screening Test,[2] the New Reynell Developmental Language Scales,[3] the British Picture Vocabulary Scales (BPVS)[4] and the Test for Reception of Grammar (TROG-2).[5] We also await the UK version of the CELF-5,[6] parts of which may be suitable.

The Computer-Based Accessible Receptive Language Assessment (CARLA)[7] is designed for children with physical disabilities, and can be used with touchscreen, switches, head-mice or eye-gaze.

The Psycholinguistic Assessments of Language Processing in Aphasia (PALPA)[8] is a battery of psycholinguistic tests to assess auditory processing, semantics, grammar, reading and spelling. Selective tests are often used with adults following head injury or stroke.

The Frenchay Screening Tool for AAC[9] is a very useful resource including sections to assess physical access, visual acuity and processing, visual contrast, symbol- or text-identification and categorisation. This may be used at this stage or later in the assessment process.

The initial Speech and Language assessment should cover the following areas, giving a detailed profile of current levels of ability.

If an Occupational Therapist is involved at this stage, then they may assess positioning, access, mounting and visual perception.

Table 10.1 Area

Area	Comments
Background Information	Including a brief developmental history, including any milestones for smiling, cooing and babbling, sitting, crawling and walking. Any diagnoses should be included. Vision and hearing, fine and gross motor skills and cognitive level, if known, should be detailed here. Sensory or behaviour issues might be explored.
Social Communication	Including use of eye contact, facial expression, body language, pointing, eye-pointing, gestures, signs, and vocalisations. It should include whether there is a clear yes/no response. It should include whether communication is pre-intentional or intentional. Communicative functions such as requesting and commenting should be explored. Repair strategies might also be explored.
Attention and Listening	Including whether there is joint attention and joint referencing. Preferred activities might be listed. An indication of how long attention to a self-chosen or adult-led task can be maintained might be useful, though this does vary enormously in clinical situations with new people.
Receptive Language	There should be informal assessment of how many information-carrying words[10] in an instruction can be understood. There might also be assessment of receptive vocabulary and/or syntax, even though standardised scores cannot be given.
Expressive Language	This should indicate how many words or signs, if any, can be used. How many information-carrying words in a phrase can be used? Any discrepancy between receptive and expressive language should be clearly stated, and this will inform any ongoing referral to an AAC Hub.
Speech Sounds	If appropriate. An inventory of meaningful sounds or words may be taken.
Literacy	Phonological or text awareness might be explored.
Educational Attainment	It may be useful to explore whether a child is keeping up with peers in the National Curriculum. Literacy and numeracy levels are helpful.
Trials of AAC	Any AAC that has been or is being tried should be detailed, including the reasons why this solution was selected at this time.

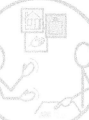

AAC may be trialled at initial assessment, or there may be subsequent sessions to try out different solutions. AAC assessment is dynamic in nature. The clinicians involved will adapt their plan as they go along, depending on how the AAC user responds. It is useful if such trials are detailed in a report, to explain why one solution was favoured over another. For example, photographs may prove more effective at this time because the child did not show recognition of symbols. A communication chart may have been chosen rather than a book because basic wants and needs are being targeted, and the child moves around a lot, so a chart is more mobile.

Following assessment, a report will be written, and an intervention plan agreed with the individual and their family. The intervention plan may include AAC alongside other interventions.

Feature-matching

In the 1990s, Shane and Costello[11] introduced a gold standard of "Feature-Mapping" to help clinicians find the best AAC solution for the client.

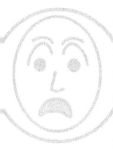

The main considerations when choosing an AAC solution are detailed in Table 10.2. It is useful to discuss these options as a team, to come up with the best solution for a potential AAC user. There may be a short list of solutions at the end of this process. In this case, the options can be trialled for a number of weeks. Hub and Spoke Services often have loan banks of equipment, as do some charitable organisations. For up-to-date information about such organisations, see http://communicationmatters.org.uk.

Table 10.2 is designed to help the Spoke Service to select appropriate no-tech, low-tech and light-tech solutions. High-tech solutions may also be considered at this stage. This might include communication apps and curriculum software on mainstream tablets and computers. Alternative access may also be necessary.

The length of the trial period will vary depending on the AAC user and the purpose of the trial. Trials of access method may be brief, to ascertain whether this piece of equipment is suitable given their visual, hearing or physical skills. Trials of AAC systems may need much longer, given that Aided Language Stimulation needs to be provided (see Chapter 9).

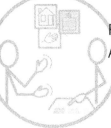

For more bespoke solutions, the Spoke Service should consider referral to a Hub AAC Service.

Table 10.2 Feature-Matching for Local Spoke AAC Service

AAC Feature	Options	Considerations
Symbolic representation	Objects Photos Symbols Words and phrases Spelling	Go for the most sophisticated option the AAC user can understand, as there is greater scope for creative communication as we progress through these options.
Symbol set	WLS PCS SymbolStix Makaton	What is used in school/college? What has been used previously? Did the AAC user show a preference?
Physical form	**Low-tech:** Single symbols Choice-board Communication chart Communication book Visual supports **Light-tech:** Single-message device Dual- or Multi-step device Multiple overlay device *MegaBee*[12] or similar **High-tech:** Communication app on tablet Communication software on a computer or dedicated AAC device	More than one of these options can be trialled. Find out what is available for loan. Refer to Regional AAC Hub following successful trials if you are considering a bespoke high-tech solution.
Keyboard options	QWERTY ABC High-frequency	Use word prediction if possible with a high-tech solution like a laptop or tablet.

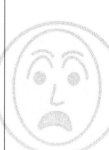

(*Continued*)

Table 10.2 Continued

AAC Feature	Options	Considerations
Vocabulary organisation	Activity-based or Category-based with core and fringe vocabulary (e.g. ACE Centre–style)[13] Pragmatic functions (e.g. PODD)	We want the present system to have the capacity to grow with the child, and have shared features with future systems so that the child does not have to relearn skills.
Screen layout	Visual Scene Display Traditional grid Combination Motor planning (e.g. LAMP)[14] Predictive grammar	Consider visual processing. Consider a trial of each.
Amount of vocabulary	How many core words? How many pages of fringe vocabulary?	Use the AAC user's current language abilities as a guide. If they are difficult to assess, start with 6–10 core words and 5–6 fringe pages.
Visual acuity and processing	Areas on page Size of symbols Space between symbols Number of symbols per page Colour contrasts Matte paper finish	May need a trial-and-error approach.
Size, weight and portability	Page or screen size Durability of materials Carry handle or strap Stand	Gauge the AAC user's needs from discussion with them and their family.

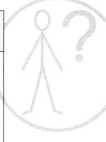

AAC Feature	Options	Considerations
Access method	**Direct:** finger-pointing (with keyguard/touchguide) fist-pointing stylus head-pointer head-mouse eye-pointing (low-tech) eye-gaze (high-tech) alternative keyboard alternative mice, e.g. trackball joystick glide-pad **Indirect:** Partner-assisted scanning Eye-pointing with coded access Type of switch Switch-scanning	Requires a joint assessment with an Occupational Therapist. May involve trials of equipment from loan bank. If eye-gaze is an option, start with eye-gaze for leisure. Liaise with your AAC Hub to discuss appropriate software and hardware options. Work on switch skills.
Mounting	Desk mount Rolling mount Wheelchair mounting Switch mounting	Requires joint assessment with an Occupational Therapist.
Personal preference	AAC user's preference Family's preference (including aesthetics and how intuitive they find the software)	Use opinion chart or rating scale. Discuss pros and cons of available options. Enable AAC user and their family to contribute to decision-making.

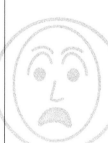

Referral to Specialised Regional AAC Assessment Hub service

Following a suitable trial period with the chosen AAC solutions, referral to the Regional Hub may be indicated. The referral criteria are shown below, taken from the current guidelines from NHS England[15] and the Communication Matters website.[16] On the following page is a decision tree, which gives a visual representation of the following referral criteria. The decision tree also shows the routes for the funding of AAC equipment, be this through the Local Spoke Service or the Regional Hub Service.

An individual who would access a specialised AAC service would have both of the following:

- A severe/complex communication difficulty associated with a range of physical, cognitive, learning or sensory deficits;

- A clear discrepancy between their level of understanding and ability to speak.

In addition, an individual must:

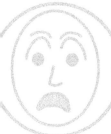

- Be able to understand the purpose of a communication aid;

- Have developed beyond cause-and-effect understanding;

and may:

- Have experience with using low-tech AAC, which is insufficient to enable them to realise their communicative potential.

The following exclusion criteria will apply to all referrals:

- Pre-verbal communication skills;

- Not having achieved cause-and-effect understanding;

- Have impaired cognitive abilities that would prevent the user from retaining information on how to use equipment.

Priority will be given to:

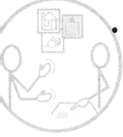

- Patients with rapidly degenerative conditions (e.g. Motor Neurone Disease); efforts will be made to ensure that these patients are assessed and/or provided with equipment as soon as practically possible.

- Patients with existing communication aid equipment that has ceased to be functional or is significantly unreliable, in order to meet their communication needs.

- Patients facing a transition to a new school/college/workplace environment or currently in a rehabilitation provision.

- Patients at risk of developing significant psychological/challenging behaviour as a consequence of their inability to communicate without a communication aid.

The Specialised AAC Assessment Hub will carry out their assessment and will share the findings and recommendations with the AAC user, their family and any professionals involved. An intervention plan will be devised, often in conjunction with an EHCP review for children and young people, to ensure that AAC contributes to long-term outcomes and that short-term targets can be reviewed.

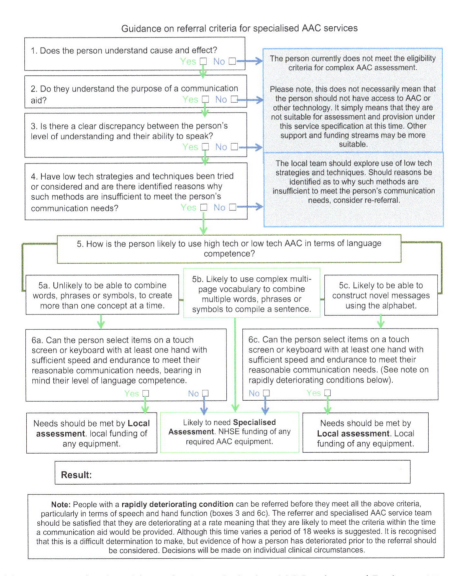

Adapted from NHS England, Guidance for Commissioning AAC Services and Equipment.[17]

Figure 10.1 Decision tree

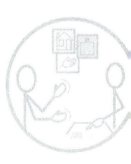

The next chapters will consider the educational settings of an AAC user, and how AAC can be implemented as part of a holistic intervention programme, to maximise the child or young person's access to education.

Notes

1 Kleiman, L. (2003) *Functional Communication Profile – Revised*. LinguiSystems.
2 http://derbyshire-language-scheme.co.uk.
3 http://reynell.glassessment.co.uk.
4 http://Gl-assessment.co.uk.
5 http://pearsonclinical.co.uk.
6 http://pearsonclinical.co.uk.
7 http://techcess.co.uk/carla/.
8 http://routledge.com.
9 http://logan-technologies.co.uk.
10 http://derbyshire-language-scheme.co.uk.
11 Shane, H. and Costello, J. (1994) *Augmentative Communication and the Feature Matching Process*. Seminar presented at the American Speech-Language-Hearing Association.
12 This is a battery-operated eye-pointing device for spelling words. See www.liberator.co.uk.
13 Latham, C. (2004) *Developing and Using a Communication Book*. Oxford: ACE Centre Advisory Trust.
14 Language Acquisition through Motor Planning. See http://liberator.co.uk.
15 http://England.nhs.uk. *Guidance for Commissioning AAC Services and Equipment*.
16 Taken from Communication Matters document, *Referral Criteria for Specialised AAC Services* (March 2016). See http://communicationmatters.org.uk.
17 www.england.nhs.uk/commissioning/wp-content/uploads/sites/12/2016/03/guid-comms-aac.pdf.

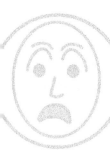

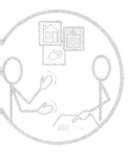

Chapter 11

Starting out with AAC

At home and in the Early Years Setting

We saw in Chapter 9 how using Aided Language Stimulation works on all levels of the Language Development Pyramid. We want to enable adults to use Aided Language Stimulation throughout the day at home and in the Early Years Setting. As we have seen, this is not that different from using typical child-directed language. We need to create a language-rich environment[1] so that there is plenty to talk about and plenty of opportunities to play, and we need to ensure there are responsive adults providing good language and AAC modelling.[2]

Home and preschool are playful settings. We want the child to explore their environment to build rich, multi-sensory experiences and connections in the brain that will support language development. So how do we do this?

Provide the same range of toys as you would any other child

In the list that follows, there are tried-and-tested favourite toys. They haven't changed much over the last 50 years. That is because they provide the child with a rich range of play experiences. There is sensorimotor or exploratory play, which makes use of the senses and movement. There is construction play, which explores concepts like object-permanence and cause-and-effect. There is messy play, which is important for learning concepts such as "dirty", "wet" and "cold". There is pretend-play, which is vital for symbolic understanding, leading to receptive language and opportunities for expressive language and developing complex narratives and social skills.

Make sure that the toys you use are accessible for the child you are working with. Consider their individual profile of physical and sensory impairments, if this is known. If the picture is still unclear, assume that the child does have some functional vision and hearing, but observe their reactions to various stimuli and note their preferences.

My favourite toys for developing communication, language and AAC skills are shown in Table 11.1. The Aided Language Stimulation ideas are not exhaustive

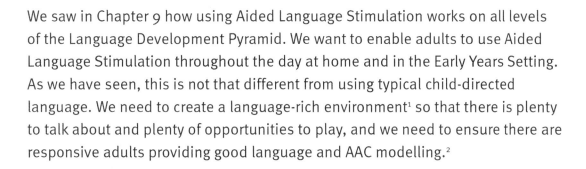

but are designed to give you a few ideas, which you can extend. See Chapter 5 for suggestions for activity-based communication boards to accompany these sets of toys. Remember to include core and fringe vocabulary, with consistent placement of core words. Alternatively, the child may have a communication book or high-tech device which includes this vocabulary. Light-tech ideas are also included: it is recommended that all settings have access to a few of these devices.[3] If you have a toy and don't have a specific communication chart made up for it, then use the core words, and point to the toy itself to build phrases. Just from the core vocabulary, you can make phrases like "you like it", "you want more", "it is mine", and "stop! No more".

Table 11.1 Toy

Toy	Adaptations	Aided Language Stimulation Ideas
Bubbles, spinners, chutes, and switch toys	Most children love bubbles being blown for them, but make sure you don't blow them in their face! You might want to introduce a switch with a bubble-machine for early switch skills. Spinners and chutes also offer anticipation for an exciting action. Other switch toys are available, e.g. cars, robots, animals.	Play "Ready, Steady, Go!" with expectant waiting for the child to indicate "Go!" with their AAC. Build phrases like "pop bubbles", "bubbles gone" and "want more bubbles". Make choices about which toy to use next, or which item to put down the chute, using AAC. Give two different commands, e.g. "go" or "stop" using light-tech or high-tech AAC. Combine two symbols with "more bubbles!" or "stop spinner" using core and fringe words.

Toy	Adaptations	Aided Language Stimulation Ideas
Balls	There is a huge variety of sizes and textures of balls available for various sensory needs. Balls with holes, ridges or soft spikes may be better for children with motor difficulties. Try a few out to see which are preferred. Light-up, noise-making and vibrating options are also available.	Play "Ready, Steady, Go!" with expectant waiting for the child to indicate "Go!" with their AAC. Make choices about who to roll the ball to next, e.g. "mummy" or "daddy" using a light-tech device. Give commands about whether you should "throw", "roll", "kick" or "catch" the ball. You could go "fast" or "slow". This could be extended with toy cars.
Musical instruments	Larger, heavier instruments may be good for sensory feedback, but smaller, lighter instruments may be easier to pick up. Have a range of auditory qualities available, e.g. low and high frequencies, loud and soft.	Play "Ready, Steady, Go!", or "go" and "stop". Give commands like "loud", "quiet", "fast" and "slow". Combine two symbols, e.g. "bang drum", "shake bells", or three symbols, e.g. "you bang tambourine", "I shake shaker". Ask "you like shaker?" or comment "you don't like drum". Describe "loud drum", "quiet xylophone".

(*Continued*)

147

Table 11.1 (Continued)

Toy	Adaptations	Aided Language Stimulation Ideas
Building blocks 	Think about size: smaller bricks are easier for children to pick up, but heavy wooden bricks provide adequate sensory feedback for children with motor impairments. Magnetic bricks can help children with physical difficulties. Blocks that light up,[4] make a noise or have interesting textures are available.	Build a tower, saying "more?" and waiting for a response. Extend this prompt to "what do we need?" modelling "more bricks!" for children ready for two-word phrases. Make choices about which colour of brick next. Give commands like "build brick!" and "knock down brick". Comment "Oh no!" or request "more!" or "again!"
Playdough	Some children might be reluctant to touch the dough, so you might need to make it very hard and dry initially: consult an Occupational Therapist if needed. Make edible dough if indicated. Move on to other messy play activities too.	Give a range of commands like "mix", "roll", "squeeze", "cut". You can try to make various foods or animals, navigating between pages in a communication book or on a high-tech device. Describe the materials, e.g. "soft", "hard". Give opinions about your creations, e.g. "I like it", "you don't [not] like it!". Build longer phrases or sentences for able AAC users.

Toy	Adaptations	Aided Language Stimulation Ideas
Doll play	A smaller doll size might work best, to allow the child to pick it up. Soft-bodied dolls are easier to cuddle, and those with heavy beans in their bottoms are easier to sit up. Make sure that your dolls reflect the diversity of your population. Wooden food may give more sensory feedback than plastic food. You could put rubber-foam tubing around the handles of cups and spoons to make them easier to pick up.	Combine core and fringe vocabulary, e.g. "help baby", "more cry[ing]". Build phrases like "baby eat", "baby sleep", "wash baby's face", "wash baby's tummy". Build longer phrases or sentences for able AAC users. Navigate between pages in a communication book or on a high-tech device, e.g. between "actions", "body-parts" and "food".
Small-world play, e.g. farm, zoo, dolls' house, garage	Large, heavy figures will provide more sensory feedback, but smaller, lighter figures may be easier for children with physical impairments to pick up. Make sure that human figures reflect the diversity of your population, including disabilities.	Program animal noises onto a light-tech device. Combine nouns and verbs to describe what figures are doing, e.g. "horse eat", "cow jump". Use adjectives, e.g. "big horse", "little horse". Navigate between pages, e.g. animals, actions, food.

In Figures 11.8–11.13 I have provided some example communication charts or pages in a communication book for the activities in Table 11.1. These will need to be adapted for the needs of individual AAC users, but may be used as a guide, or for general AAC resources in the Early Years Setting. The core words might be worn on an apron or key-ring by adults, so that they are always accessible. This layout is taken from ACE Centre communication books.[5]

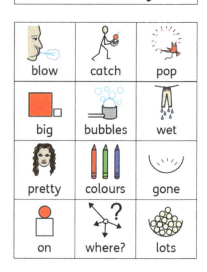

Figure 11.8 Core words bubble play

Widgit Symbols © Widgit Software 2002–2017 www.widgit.com

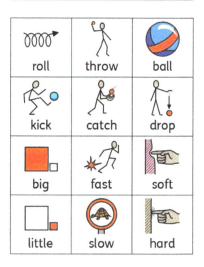

Figure 11.9 Core words ball play

Widgit Symbols © Widgit Software 2002–2017 www.widgit.com

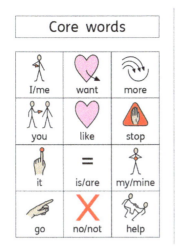
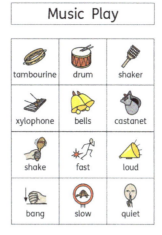

Figure 11.10 Core words music play

Widgit Symbols © Widgit Software 2002–2017 www.widgit.com

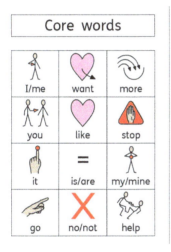
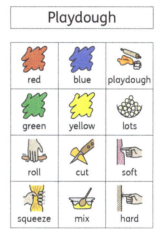
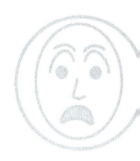

Figure 11.11 Core words playdough

Widgit Symbols © Widgit Software 2002–2017 www.widgit.com

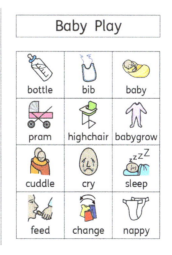
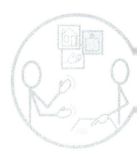

Figure 11.12 Core words baby play

Widgit Symbols © Widgit Software 2002–2017 www.widgit.com

Core words		
I/me	want	more
you	like	stop
it	is/are	my/mine
go	no/not	help

Farm Animals		
horse	cow	sheep
pig	chicken	duck
eat	climb	naughty
jump	run	dirty

Figure 11.13 Core words farm animals

Widgit Symbols © Widgit Software 2002–2017 www.widgit.com

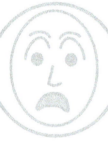

Provide a communication-friendly environment[6]

We want to immerse children in language and AAC, so that it is part of everything we do. I will now consider rooms in the house and then areas in a nursery setting, and how we can set up the environment to support communication.

General principles of communication-friendly environments:

- Reduce distractions. Turn the TV or radio off. Hide your phone.

- Don't have too many choices of toys out at any one time.

- Make the shared activity the most interesting thing in the room.

- Position yourself where your child can easily make eye contact.

- Have AAC in an accessible position too.

- Think about what AAC or visual support you need in each area.

- Have a special quiet area where you can share books.

- You might want to set aside "Special Time" with each of your children for 10 minutes each day. Try to give them your undivided attention at this time.

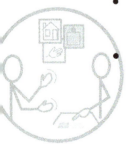

- Slow down. We all tend to be in a rush, which doesn't leave time for children to think, and wonder, and talk.

- Restrict screen time from a young age. One hour per day is recommended. This allows children all the multi-sensory, physical, social, creative and imaginative play time they need.

AAC in different areas of the house

Because this section mentions communication charts a lot, I would just like to revisit communication charts. It is recommended that communication charts have a combination of core and fringe vocabulary, and that as much as possible there is consistent placement of the core vocabulary across different communication charts.

One solution is to combine a core communication chart with various communication charts of fringe vocabulary. The core communication chart travels around the house, whilst the fringe charts tend to stay near the things they refer to. Note that the core words are positioned as much as possible in the order they are used to make a phrase. This introduces the idea from early on that we read from left to right.

I'm not suggesting that every child should have every AAC resource mentioned here. These are ideas only and can be selected as appropriate.

Table 11.2 Rooms of house

Bedroom	<ul><li>Label your child's drawers and wardrobe in the symbols for the clothes that go there.</li><li>Have communication charts or pages in a communication book for "Getting Dressed" and "Weather" so that you can match clothes with the weather today.</li><li>Have communication charts or pages in a communication books for various play activities (see the examples earlier in this chapter).</li><li>Have a choice-board of clothes, or a visual sequence showing what your child needs to put on and take off every day. These could be Velcroed, so that they can be changed to suit the weather.</li><li>Label your child's toy box or cupboard with the toys that are kept there.</li><li>Have a light-tech device by the bed that says a fun message like "wakey wakey!" or "night night, sweet dreams!"</li></ul>

(Continued)

Table 11.2 (Continued)

Bathroom	<ul><li>Have a light-tech device mounted near the bathroom door that says "I need the toilet!"</li><li>Have a laminated communication chart that can be used in the bath. This might be stuck to a swimming float. Bath-time is a brilliant time to talk about parts of the body, verbs like "wash" and "splash", and adjectives like "dirty" and "wet".</li></ul>
Kitchen	<ul><li>Label the fridge and cupboards with symbols for items that are kept there.</li><li>Have a dual-message device that is programmed with "yummy" and "yucky" so that you can talk about food!</li><li>Have a communication chart or a page in a communication book for mealtimes.</li></ul>
Lounge	<ul><li>Have communication charts or pages in a communication book for book-reading, singing songs, or watching TV and DVDs.</li><li>Have communication charts of pages in a communication book for various play activities (see examples earlier in this chapter).</li><li>You might want a special communication chart or light-tech device with instructions like "change the channel" and "turn it up". Or you might not!</li></ul>
Garden or Park	<ul><li>A core vocabulary communication chart or key-ring of symbols might be attached to the buggy. "Go" and "stop" are useful for play equipment.</li><li>Have a communication chart or pages in a communication book for the things you can see and do in your garden, or in the park.</li></ul>
Car or Bus	<ul><li>A light-tech device that says a fun phrase like "beep beep" or "go faster!" might be mounted on your child's car seat.</li><li>Have a communication chart or key-ring of fringe vocabulary of things you can see from the bus or car.</li></ul>

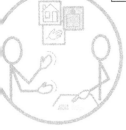

Table 11.3 AAC in different areas of the Early Years Setting

Carpet Area	• Have comfortable seating in this area, and make sure that the AAC user is at the same level as their peers, to enable easy interaction. • Make sure that any books or interesting displays are also accessible to the AAC user. • This area lends itself to shared visual supports for registration time. These might include: a days of the week chart with weather symbols that can be removed; a simple visual timetable; behaviour supports such as traffic lights or reminders for good sitting and looking.[7] • Have a core vocabulary communication chart within easy reach at all times. Some settings decide that staff are going to wear an apron with core vocabulary always visible.
Bathroom	• Have a light-tech device mounted near the bathroom door that says "I need the toilet!" or "wash your hands!" • Have a laminated communication chart that can be used in the wash-basins. This can include verbs like "wash" and "dry" "splash", and adjectives like "dirty", "clean", "wet" and "dry".
Construction Area	• Have a communication chart for brick play that can be used with lots of different types of construction toys, e.g. wooden blocks, magnetic blocks, Duplo. • Have a light-tech dual message or multi-step device that says "build it up" and "knock it down!".
Home Corner	• Think about how you make resources accessible. If the AAC user needs to have time in a standing frame, then they might do this in the home corner, and access the toy cooker and sink at this time. • Have symbolised visual supports like shopping lists or recipe cards. • At times when your home corner is converted into a shop, café or office, change the symbolised visual supports to match. Try not to be too noun-based, but think about verbs, adjectives and social phrases too. • Have a light-tech device with fun recorded messages like "cup of tea please!" or if it is a shop "next please" or if it is a café "waiter!" • Have core and fringe communication charts to suit the resources on offer.

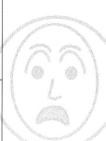

(*Continued*)

Table 11.3 (Continued)

Art and Craft Area	• Have core and fringe communication charts available. The fringe communication chart could be suitable for a range of art and craft materials, with verbs like "cut", "stick", "tear" and "paint", and adjectives like "sparkly", "spotty" and "stripy". • An opinions chart may be useful here too, e.g. "I think it is . . ." + "beautiful"
Book Area	• You might have communication charts for book-reading, people games or singing songs in here. • Have a range of different types of books that are accessible for the AAC user. Thickened pages are often easier to handle. Those with holes and flaps are fun. Include tactile books. See Table 11.4 for more ideas.
Outdoor Area	• Encourage peers to play cooperatively, giving instructions like "go", "stop" and "more" with the core vocabulary communication chart when on bikes and swings. • You might want a fringe communication chart for the things you can see and do in the outdoor area. • Have a light – tech device to say "can I have a turn?" and use sand-timers to encourage children to wait for their turn. • This is an area where there tends to be a lot of conflict, and so a visual support with social phrases might be helpful, e.g. "sorry", "can I play?"

I deliberately haven't included snack-time in the table, as this is typically a time when AAC is used quite well. However, the danger is that snack-time is the *only* time AAC is used. If a child is only using their AAC for 10 minutes per day, 5 days a week, it will take them 80 years to reach the language competence of a typical 3-year-old.[8] To give AAC users the same language stimulation as their talking peers, we need to immerse them in AAC throughout the day!

Book-sharing and AAC

Enjoying books should be part of every child's experience. Book-sharing with a responsive adult works on all parts of the Language Development Pyramid. Sharing books offers a special time where a child can slow down and their non-verbal reactions to pictures and words can really be noticed.

You don't have to read a book from cover to cover to enjoy it: let the child lead at first, and then they will want to read whole stories later. Sharing two or three books

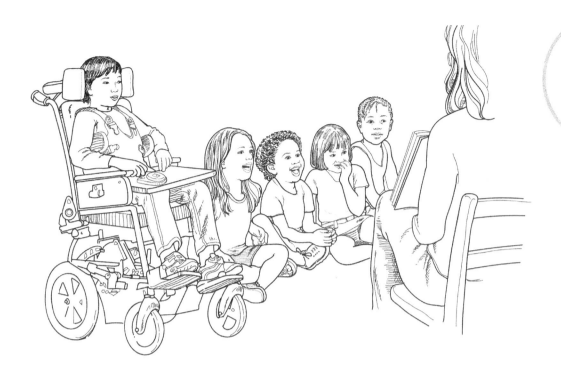

per day will provide children with richer vocabularies, an instinct for grammar and syntax, and an interest in the rhythm and sound of spoken language. This will increase their readiness for school and literacy.

Many typically developing children go through a phase of wanting to hear the same favourite book at least once per day. We need to give AAC users the opportunity to also go through this stage. It is the repetition of such texts that contributes to a child's familiarity and comfort in reading, and in developing memory for phrases and text. Be alert to signs that an AAC user has a favourite book, and make sure that they have a way of requesting it.

I would recommend that you use real books. Books are multi-sensory, beautiful objects. We can poke our fingers into holes in the page, and lift up flaps. There is a delight in turning a page, and seeing what happens next. Real books invite close attention and slowing down to absorb information.

To promote use of AAC communication when sharing books, Kent-Walsh et al.[9] recommend using a structure that they call RAA RAA RAA. This stands for "Read, Ask, Answer": read some of the text, ask an open-ended (wh-) question and model the answer using AAC.

Table 11.4 displays ideas for reading books in a small group with an AAC user. It is likely that all the children in the group will want to use AAC resources, including speaking children. This is fine, as it provides modelling for the AAC user, and shows that AAC communication has a valued place in the social world.

Table 11.4 Different books

Dear Zoo Rod Campbell (Macmillan)	Programme the phrase "I sent him back" onto a light-tech device. Have animal symbols available to match with the pictures in the book. Use core vocabulary to comment on the animals, e.g. "I like it", "I want it", "it is mine", "no, stop, go!"
Peepo Janet and Allan Ahlberg (Puffin)	Programme "Here's a little baby, one, two, three. . ." and "Peepo!" onto a light-tech device. Use symbols to spot the named items, e.g. teddy, ball, doll, dog (they appear repeatedly).
Here Come the Babies Catherine and Lawrence Anholt (Walker Books)	This is the best book ever for modelling two-word phrases. Model phrases like "baby crying", "baby eating", "baby happy", "baby sad".
We're Going on a Bear Hunt Michael Rosen and Helen Oxenbury (Walker Books)	Programme "we're going on a bear hunt", "we can't go over it", "we can't go under it", on a sequenced message device or onto single-message devices for different children to press in a group reading. Talk about concepts like "wet" and "dirty" and "cold".
The Very Hungry Caterpillar Eric Carle (Puffin)	Match food symbols to the foods that the caterpillar is eating. Children could suggest other foods the caterpillar might eat, using AAC. These could be silly! Model the phrase "caterpillar's eating. . ." for the child to complete. Describe the caterpillar and the butterfly using describing symbols.

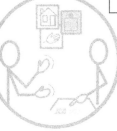

Farmer Duck Martin Waddell and Helen Oxenbury (Walker Books)	Programme a light-tech device with the animal noises, and the refrain of "How goes the work?" Match farm animal symbols with pictures in the book. Model two-word and three-word phrases like "farmer [in] bed", "duck [in] snow", "duck digging", "duck washing", "duck sad".
Handa's Surprise Eileen Browne (Walker Books)	Programme "I wonder which fruit Handa will like the best?" onto a light-tech device. Match fruit and animal symbols with pictures in the book. Just like Here Come the Babies is brilliant for two-word phrases, this book is brilliant for three-word phrases. Model three-word phrases like "zebra eat orange" and "elephant eat mango".
The Tiger Who Came to Tea Judith Kerr (HarperCollins)	Programme a light-tech device with eating noises that a child can activate every time in the story the tiger eats or drinks something. Match "food" and "kitchen equipment" symbols to the pictures in the book. Model combining core words with fringe words like "more biscuit", "more cake" and "no food", "no water". Model three-word phrases like "tiger eating sandwich", "tiger drinking tea".
Cockatoos Quentin Blake (Red Fox)	Programme a light-tech device with "Good Morning my fine feathered friends!" Use "position" symbols and "furniture" and other symbols to say where the cockatoos are hiding, e.g. "in flower", "on chair". Use a visual support with numbers to count the cockatoos on each page.

(Continued)

Table 11.4 (Continued)

Eat Your Peas Kes Gray and Nick Sharratt (Red Fox)	Programme a light-tech device with the refrain "I don't like peas". Use the "food", "places" and "transport" pages of a communication book or a light-tech or high-tech device to talk about what Daisy's mum will buy her if she eats her peas. Talk about what you might ask for, or about food you don't like.
You Choose Pippa Goodhart and Nick Sharratt (Picture Corgi)	This is the most fantastic book for exploring pages of vocabulary in a communication book or on a high-tech device. Categories include "clothes", "animals", "transport", "food", "furniture", "jobs" and "activities". Use a "describing" page or an "opinions" page to comment on the pictures. You could use the book as inspiration for story-building on a light- or high-tech device.

Access to the alphabet

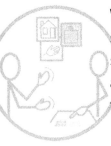

Once a child has started their early years education, they will be exposed to the alphabet. It is important that the child using AAC has access to this too. This may take the form of a low-tech alphabet chart. Assuming that the child will move on to a QWERTY keyboard in school, this layout is generally preferred, so that the child will not have to relearn a different layout later. However there may be individual reasons why an ABC or high-frequency layout is preferred. Vowels and consonants may be colour-coded. Lowercase is generally preferred by teachers.

It is important that adults model the use of letters and their sounds. They might start by drawing attention to the initial letter and sound of the child's name. This might be extended to find other everyday words beginning with this letter or sound. A book might even be created.

When other children are exposed to the alphabet, through songs, books or structured activities, the AAC user should have access to their alphabet AAC. Adults should model the sound and letter of focus, using the child's AAC. For example, if an alphabet book is being read (I love *Quentin Blake's ABC*),[10] the adult can point to the relevant letter and make its sound or say its name.

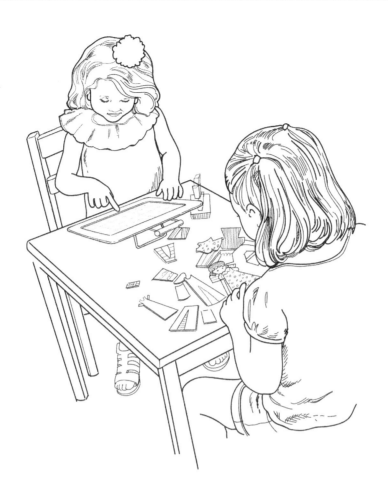

There is currently some disagreement about whether to focus on the letter sound or name first. In the UK, the letter sound tends to be taught first. It is recommended that practitioners keep up to date with current research and early years curriculum guidance. It is important to discuss and agree on the method to be used as a team, so that all those modelling to the AAC user are consistent in their approach.

A waiting game

AAC has been introduced, and all the adults are desperate for the child to use it. Sometimes the adults are disappointed when the child doesn't start responding by using the AAC straight away.

Be patient! Remember how long we have to model spoken language to a typically developing child before we get anything back? A year. How long does it take for a typically developing child to reach language competence? Five years. If a child has a developmental delay, then they are likely to need longer and need more repetition.

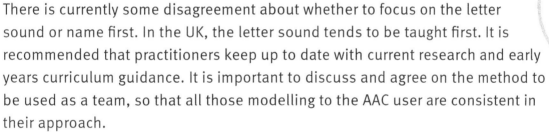

Just carry on with the Aided Language Stimulation all day and every day, little and often. Don't give up!

Cues and prompts

That is not to say that we don't use any cues or prompts. Cues are environmental. For example if a child has a switch to activate a bubble machine, then the cue might be that the bubbles have stopped. Prompts come from a communication partner. They can be:

- Expectant waiting: leaning forward, eye-pointing at the switch.

- A gesture or a point towards the switch.

- A verbal prompt. Saying "oh no! bubbles stopped!" or "more bubbles?" Avoid saying "press the switch": we don't want the child to be passive and waiting for an instruction to press the switch. Instead we want them to actively recognise a need, and realise they can do something.

- A touch to their hand to remind them they can do something.

- Hand-under-hand[11] support to press the switch.

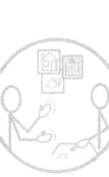

We don't want the child to be prompt-dependent, so we will try the prompt with the least amount of support from us first, starting at the top of this list, and working our way down. Some types of prompts may work best with a child, and this can be noted for all who work with them.

Response time

Children need longer than adults to process spoken language. If a child has additional cognitive, physical, sensory, language or social communication needs, we may need to give them a little bit longer. Get to know the child you are working with. Experiment with leaving a longer gap than feels comfortable. A child's processing of language may vary across different settings. Reduce background noise and distractions, and make sure that the child is not expending unnecessary energy on maintaining their position or accessing resources. This will all help with freeing up processing for communication.

The importance of talking nonsense

All children talk nonsense. It is their birthright. Children love playing with the sound of words, using new and funny words, and making absurd sentences. It is one of the ways they learn about the structure of language. When a child gets a new AAC device, particularly a high-tech VOCA, adults around them often express concern that the child is just talking nonsense. Some children have favourite pages or phrases that they return to and repeat endlessly. It is important to provide reassurance here. The child is experimenting with their new voice. Often children will press buttons to listen to the different words on their device. They will create great long strings of apparently meaningless repetitive babble. This is what typically developing children have been able to do from babyhood, so the AAC user is catching up!

Whilst this babble stage may be annoying, NEVER turn the volume off on a VOCA. You would not tape up a speaking child's mouth, so it is just not acceptable to take away a VOCA user's voice. They, like all other children, have to learn when it is OK to talk loudly, be rude and talk nonsense, and when it is not. This might take a while. Give them an outlet for silliness, and allow extra time for this if the VOCA is new. Remind them to be quiet at key times for short periods, but let them keep their VOCA with the volume up.

Which skills to work on?

As we have acknowledged in Chapter 7, AAC is complicated. We need to work on a number of skills concurrently. At this time when a child has just been introduced to their AAC system, they might be working on cognitive skills like cause and effect. They might be working on social communication skills like initiating. They might be developing gross motor skills like core stability for sitting, and fine motor skills like pressing and releasing a switch. They might be fine-tuning sensory skills, like tracking a moving object or locating a sound. They might be working on language skills like matching a symbol with an object. They might be working on strategic skills like a consistent yes/no response.

We need to keep all of these skills moving on, because they will be important for the future. The AAC solution that the child has now will not be the AAC solution they have for life. It will evolve over time as the child's skills develop. I am going to represent these concurrent skills developing as the "AAC Therapy Pie".

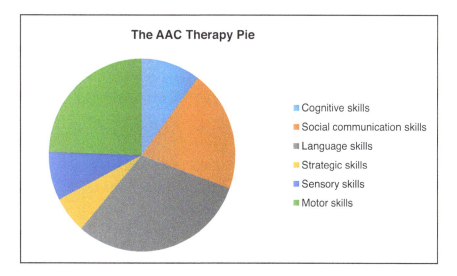

Figure 11.14 AAC Therapy Pie

The proportions of the different elements will vary over time. AAC is a collection of many different skill areas, and these are prioritised differently at various life stages. Many professionals will need to coordinate their intervention plan to be working towards the common goal of AAC competence. The multidisciplinary team will vary with each child, but is likely to include a Paediatrician, Physiotherapist, Occupational Therapist and Speech and Language Therapist. Depending on Local Service Provision, there may be an Early Support Coordinator, Portage Worker, Hearing Impairment or Visual Impairment Specialist too. If the family has engaged any independent therapists, then they also need to be working towards the common goal of AAC competence.[12] Each profession will have other concerns too: for example, the Paediatrician may be managing epilepsy or sleep; the Physiotherapist will be concerned with mobility, the Occupational Therapist may be assessing the home for adaptations, and the Speech and Language Therapist may be managing eating and drinking. Regular Multi-Disciplinary Meetings should be prioritised so that all those involved have a shared understanding of the holistic needs of the child.

Monitoring progress

Targets are likely to be part of the therapy process. See Chapter 16 for more information about this. In terms of recording what a child is doing right now with their AAC system, two tools are invaluable. One is to take regular video recordings. The way that these are stored will need careful consideration, to comply with data protection. It may be that they are used to transcribe what a child has done and then are deleted. Don't use personal devices such as smartphones for this purpose: data is kept for a period of time and may be shared with your iCloud or Dropbox, which would be a breach of data protection. Therefore use recording devices provided for this professional purpose.

Transcriptions of AAC

You may watch the video and transcribe what the child has done in detail, using a form similar to that included at the end of this chapter. These record sheets will be invaluable for the Speech and Language Therapist to track vocabulary, syntax and pragmatic functions. They will also contain information about access method.

A more informal approach, and one that I strongly recommend, is having a small notebook that travels around with the child in their AAC bag, and the things that the child has said are noted, verbatim. Of course there are privacy issues here as well: these should be discussed with the family, and the book should be used sensitively. But again, this gives a really quick reference about the vocabulary, syntax and pragmatic functions that are being used on a day-to-day basis.

The following conventions are used for transcriptions of AAC communication in printed publications:[13]

Table 11.5 AAC Transcription Record Sheet

Child's Name:	Transcription Conventions:
Date of Birth:	Spoken utterance (sp)
NHS Number:	Spoken utterances on a voice-output AAC device (vo)
	Quick phrases (vo)
	Signs (M) for Makaton. Indicate sign boundaries with a dash.
	Symbols (WLS) (PCS) (SS) for SymbolStix. Also use a dash.
	s-p-e-lling (p) with prediction
	(The communication partner's turns)
	Prompt (p)

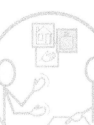

Date	Where Who Why	What the child said and did (+ what the adult said and did)

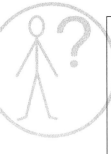

> *Spoken utterances are italicised*
>
> *'Spoken utterances on a voice-output AAC device are italicised and in quotation marks'*
>
> SIGNS ARE IN CAPITALS
>
> *SYMBOLS ARE IN ITALICISED CAPITALS*
>
> <u>Quick phrases that have been programmed onto a device are underlined</u>
>
> *s-p-e-lling (p)* is underlined with hyphens between letters. If prediction is used from there, I suggest that this can be indicated with (p).

However, with most people's handwriting it is difficult to italicise. I would therefore suggest brackets to indicate the mode of communication:

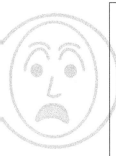

> Spoken utterance (sp)
>
> Spoken utterances on a voice-output AAC device (vo)
>
> Quick phrases can be underlined (vo)
>
> Signs (M) for Makaton; (SA) for Signalong. Indicate sign boundaries with a – or +.
>
> Symbols (WLS) (PCS) (SS) for SymbolStix. Indicate symbol boundaries with a – or +.
>
> *s-p-e-lling (p)* is underlined with hyphens between letters. If prediction is used from there, I suggest that this can be indicated with (p).
>
> (The communication partner's turns can be in brackets)
>
> Prompt (p)

I would suggest that you stick a copy of this table in the front of the exercise book, deleting any methods that are not used by the child.

Support for families

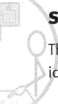

This chapter has largely focused on the Early Years Setting, though many of the ideas for play and sharing books are relevant for home. It is important that parents and siblings continue to use the child's AAC system in everyday routines and play, continuing the Aided Language Stimulation techniques from the last chapter.

The introduction of AAC to family life has a dramatic impact. Parents report that they initially feel that their successful unaided communication methods with their child are being undermined or devalued when AAC is proposed. Parents are often going through a period of adjustment to their child's diagnosis and can be overwhelmed by incoming information. AAC adds another burden to a busy schedule of therapy and medical appointments. However, parents also report that it can be a struggle to get AAC support for their child. They often have to become "pushy parents" to get AAC assessment.

Families of AAC users often report that they operate strongly as a family team around the child who uses AAC. Older siblings tend to be protective of their sibling who uses AAC, whilst younger siblings often take on the role of interpreter. Siblings often facilitate communication with wider family members like grandparents, who may be less familiar with AAC.[14] Mothers tend to take on the role of being their child's advocate and coordinating AAC intervention. There is a shift in family roles that can affect all family members.[15]

However, families also report that they feel isolated from wider society. When out and about, other peoples' curiosity about their child's AAC system can become intrusive. Families report that they enjoy spending time with other families of AAC users, because they have shared experiences. This is not always easy, given the relatively low numbers of AAC users, and especially of high-tech AAC users.

AAC Hubs and national organisations such as Communication Matters[16] and 1Voice[17] have a part to play here. Social events for AAC users and their families are a valuable way of connecting with other families in a similar situation. There may be holiday programmes for AAC users and their siblings, or days out for the whole family. The ultimate aim might be for the service-users to take ownership of the network, and independently coordinate events.

You Matter is a formal course for family members and teaching staff. This has been developed collaboratively by Specialised AAC Centres and available for services to purchase.[18] It is a course run over eight sessions, including information about AAC, exploring personal experiences, offering practice in using AAC more effectively (including optional video feedback) and developing the AAC system further, through making low-tech AAC resources or programming the high-tech device.

Kent and Medway Communication and Assistive Technology (CAT) Service offer an informal rolling programme of support sessions to the families of AAC users, called

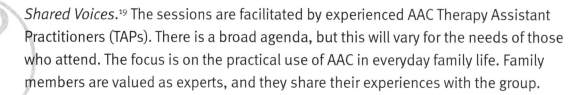

Shared Voices.[19] The sessions are facilitated by experienced AAC Therapy Assistant Practitioners (TAPs). There is a broad agenda, but this will vary for the needs of those who attend. The focus is on the practical use of AAC in everyday family life. Family members are valued as experts, and they share their experiences with the group.

The Therapy Assistant Practitioners provide family members with an AAC device that is the same as their child's, including the child's vocabulary package, for each session. This allows family members to practice using the device without depriving their child of their own for the session.

The *Shared Voices* group often feeds back family experiences to the CAT Team, in order to inform best practice when working with families.

The format of *Shared Voices* changes slightly with every cycle, dependent on the needs of the participants. Table 11.6 contains a sample plan of four sessions in a *Shared Voices* cycle.[20] Each week there is an overall theme. The themed activity provides a fun and practical way to explore this.

Table 11.6 Shared Voices Agenda

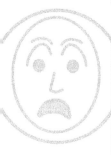

Session One: Time to Explore

1 Meet and greet: tea and coffee; brief introductions.
 2 Ice-breaker: Hand out *M&Ms* or *Smarties*.
  • Red – Something funny your child does
  • Blue – Your favourite food
  • Yellow – Your favourite film/book
  • Green – Your child's favourite film/book/toy
  • Orange – What did you do last night?
  • Brown – Something you enjoy doing with your child/children
 3 Themed Vocabulary Activity. Using picture cards, ask the parent/carer to find the item within their child's vocabulary package. Start with an easier item like an animal or transport item to build confidence. Talk about whether items are where they would expect to find them. Talk about how they are feeling as they search. Remember, this week is about getting hands on, feeling the fear and surviving!
 4 Feedback from group: General chat around the session, if it was what they had expected. Talk about upcoming weeks and themes, ask for suggestions of things they want covered.
 5 Homework: Come next week with video footage/photo of child on their phone to enable the group to put a face to a name.

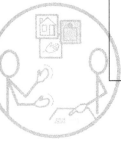

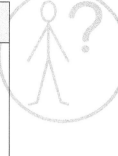

Session 2: Real Life

1 Meet and greet: tea and coffee. Share photo or video of their child (homework) and any news since last session. Emphasis on learning from each other; support each person to feel valued; give time to feed back to group. Open questions from TAPs to tease out any worries there may be.

2 Ice-breaker: The Wool Game. Someone starts with ball of wool and talks about something they like to do. If anyone in the group shares this interest, then the wool is passed to them whilst holding on to the end of the wool. This continues on until you can see that the whole group is connected in some way.

3 Themed Vocabulary activity: Recap last week's activity. This week the picture cards show more difficult items such as "umbrella". If the word is not on the device, then the parent/carers try to describe it.

The theme for today is "real life situations". Families often feel that they don't need to use AAC devices because they know what their child is saying or can interpret accurately what they need. However communication is not about just here and now but about the future. Brainstorm together reasons to communicate and get them to give examples of each, using devices:

- Asking questions
- Greeting friends and family
- Commenting
- Expressing likes/dislikes
- Indicating a problem
- Complaining
- Indicating a preference
- Making requests
- Giving instructions to a family member
- Talking about what they have done at school
- Making up funny stories
- Telling jokes
- Pretending.

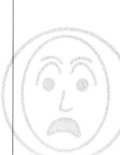

Discuss how to incorporate AAC into the daily routine, from getting up to going to bed. How to manage time with siblings. How to encourage the wider family to use AAC.

4 Feedback from the group about today's session.

5 Homework. Come next week with something that your child likes (toy/book/game/app).

(Continued)

Table 11.6 (Continued)

Session 3: Motivation

1 Meet and greet: tea and coffee. Share news since last session. What's going well and not so well. Encourage parent/carers to support one another and to come up with ideas together. Emphasis on learning from each other; support each person so that they feel valued.

2 Ice-breaker: Dice Game. Roll the dice that the number corresponds to:
  - Something you can't live without.
  - Something your child does that makes you smile.
  - Your favourite holiday.
  - Your child's favourite activity to do with you.
  - Your favourite song.
  - Your child's favourite item.

3 Themed activity: Motivation: discuss what they have bought (something their child likes). How can they use this alongside the device? Encourage other parents to come up with ideas. Time to explore the devices.

4 Describing game: A jar with random treasures inside (e.g. costume jewellery, a worry doll, a shell, a friendship bracelet, cracker toys, party favours) is passed around. Parents describe one of the objects using their child's device. Share further ideas of how to use the device creatively when you can't find a word.

5 Feedback from the group about today's session: How do they feel about using the device. Are we covering everything? Any questions?

6 Homework: Come next week with a resource they have found useful, e.g. website, book. Share emails?

Session 4: Fun, Fun, Fun!

1 Meet and greet: tea and coffee. Share news since last session. Homework review: sharing resources/websites. Give time to chat.

2 Ice-breaker: Simon Says using devices. Be as silly as you like.

3 Themed activity. Fun games on devices. Share games, apps, etc. Allow parents to lead more this week, giving the sense that they are now the experts.

4 Feedback from the group about today's session: Reflections on what has been learnt over the last three sessions: What have they found out about themselves? Any skills they didn't know they had? Impact on wider family? How to take this forward? How might the group stay in touch?

5 Feedback forms.

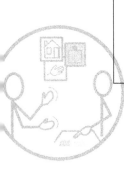

The Early Years Foundation Stage Profile (EYFSP)[21]

By the end of the Early Years Foundation Stage (the end of the reception year), the school must complete the Early Years Foundation Stage Profile (EYFSP). This shows the child's progress in relation to 17 Early Learning Goals. The three levels are at the *Expected* level, at an *Emerging* level, or *Exceeding* the level. This is a summative judgement for each Early Learning Goal, based on evidence of learning collected over the EYFS.

There is no requirement for how settings collect evidence. Evidence may include informal observation, video recording, photographs, samples of work, the child's view and information from parents and professionals. Therefore information from AAC targets and AAC transcriptions is valid. It is important that professionals do not see this process as a box-ticking process, but collect qualitative information that will inform the next steps. Another trap is to assume that a child who does not use speech cannot achieve some of these targets: as the following examples show, other modes of communication can be used.

For those children who are at an *Emerging* level, settings should provide more detailed information about a child's profile of needs, to ensure adequate transition planning for the child's needs in Year 1.

On the following page is an example of a profile for two very different AAC users.

Sam is likely to receive a diagnosis of Autism Spectrum Condition. He understands some spoken words if they are accompanied by signs or symbols. His communication is by non-verbal means, like proximity, body movements, reaching or pulling someone's hand to reach for something, and vocalising. He is being encouraged to make choices from a choice-board and use visual supports for his behaviour and learning. He is largely at the Emerging level, with strengths in physical and computer skills.

Aisha has four-limb Cerebral Palsy. She has unimpaired cognitive functioning. There may be some visual processing difficulties and a mild-moderate hearing loss. She has a PEG feeding tube. Aisha struggles with all aspects of fine and gross motor control. She uses wheelchair and a walker. Aisha is learning how to use switches and eye-gaze to access her high-tech communication device. Aisha is largely at the Expected level, with adaptations having being made for her physical difficulties.

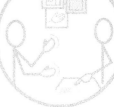

Table 11.7 EYFS Profile for Two AAC Users

Area of Learning	Early Learning Goal (ELG)	Sam	Aisha
Communication and language	**1. Listening and attention** Children listen attentively in a range of situations. They listen to stories, accurately anticipating key events and respond to what they hear with relevant comments, questions or actions. They give their attention to what others say and respond appropriately, while engaged in another activity.	**Emerging** Sam explored a tactile book, putting his fingers on the bumpy and crinkly textures. Sam engaged for 2 minutes with sensory toys, including the vibrating ball and snake, and the light strands. Sam banged and shook musical instruments. He smiled when an adult joined in.	**Expected** Aisha listened attentively at story-time, and used a light-tech device to contribute a repeated refrain in *We're Going on a Bear Hunt*. Aisha did not need prompting to activate her device at the right time, because she was keeping track of the story. Aisha used her talker to say what else the caterpillar might eat in *The Very Hungry Caterpillar*.

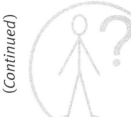

	Emerging	Expected
2. Understanding Children follow instructions involving several ideas or actions. They answer "how" and "why" questions about their experiences and in response to stories or events.	**Emerging** Sam followed a "now and next" board to finish building a tower before going outside. Sam got his coat when I said and signed "coat". When Sam was offered a choice of "car" or "ball" on a choice-board, Sam touched the "car" symbol.	**Expected** Aisha sequenced instructions to make a recipe book for making pancakes, including "add the flour", "mix in the egg" and "pour in milk". I asked Aisha why she thought Elmer was sad in the story. Aisha said "no friend" and made a sad face.
3. Speaking Children express themselves effectively, showing awareness of listeners' needs. They use past, present and future forms accurately when talking about events that have happened or are to happen in the future. They develop their own narratives and explanations by connecting ideas or events.	**Emerging** Sam took me by the arm to the shelf where we keep Duplo. Sam pulled my arm to the box. I said, "you want Duplo?" Sam vocalised to indicate "yes". Sam brought in some photos of his trip to LEGOLAND. He smiled and rocked happily in his seat when I pointed to the photos and commented on them. We added a symbol sentence to each photo and stuck them in a photo book.	**Expected** Aisha said "I go grandma" on her talker. I said "you're going to your Grandma's?" Aisha shook her head. I said "you went to your Grandma's?" Aisha nodded. We composed a joint story using Aisha's talker. Aisha took turns with her friend to add words to the story. Aisha added characters, places, actions and objects, in response to *Who, where, what doing and with what* questions.

(Continued)

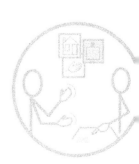

Table 11.7 (Continued)

Area of Learning	Early Learning Goal (ELG)	Sam	Aisha
Physical development	**4. Moving and handling Children** show good control and co-ordination in large and small movements. They move confidently in a range of ways, safely negotiating space. They handle equipment and tools effectively, including pencils for writing.	**Emerging** Sam brought in a Transformer toy from home and showed the group how to change it from a robot to a car. Sam climbed to the top of the climbing frame in the outdoor space. He waited for his turn before going down the slide. Sam does not show interest in holding pencils or crayons yet.	**Emerging** Aisha used a switch to play a BigBang computer game. She showed good "press-and-hold" skills. Aisha used her walker to move from the home corner to the construction area, stopping to let another child move out of the way. Aisha put her hand in paint and made marks with her whole hand on paper.
	5. Health and self-care Children know the importance for good health of physical exercise, and a healthy diet, and talk about ways to keep healthy and safe. They manage their own basic hygiene and personal needs successfully, including dressing and going to the toilet independently.	**Emerging** Sam used a visual schedule with prompts to follow each step in turn when washing and drying his hands. Sam touched a piece of apple and poked a piece of banana with a spoon at snack time. He was rewarded with a *wotsit*.	**Expected** Aisha indicated that I had not connected her feeding tube properly by vocalising and wriggling. Aisha was happy to sit on her new toilet seat before lunch. Aisha helped me to put her coat on by holding out the correct arm in turn.

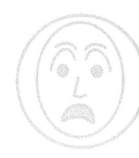

Personal, social and emotional development	6. Self-confidence and self-awareness	Emerging	Expected
	Children are confident to try new activities and say why they like some activities more than others. They are confident to speak in a familiar group, will talk about their ideas, and will choose the resources they need for their chosen activities. They say when they do or don't need help.	Sam tolerated another child sharing his space in the construction area for 2 minutes. Sam took three turns with the other child adding a brick to a tower. Sam then moved away. Sam accepted when the sand-timer ran out and it was time to stop playing on the computer. When I asked if Sam wanted me to blow bubbles, he bounced on his toes. Sam waited for me to blow bubbles and popped them. Sam did not want to blow bubbles himself.	Aisha chose "messy play" using a choice-board. She put her hands into the cornflour and indicated which materials to add, including food-colouring and glitter. Aisha said "fun" on her talker when I asked her what she thought of the activity later on. Aisha told the group about her new puppy, using the news page on her talker. She answered questions about her puppy, like what he eats and what he plays with.

(Continued)

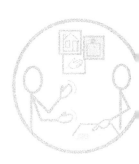

Table 11.7 (Continued)

Area of Learning	Early Learning Goal (ELG)	Sam	Aisha
	7. Managing feelings and behaviour Children talk about how they and others show feelings, talk about their own and others' behaviour, and its consequences, and know that some behaviour is unacceptable. They work as part of a group or class, and understand and follow the rules. They adjust their behaviour to different situations, and take changes of routine in their stride.	**Emerging** Sam looked at and listened to his visual social story about taking turns. He then took three turns with a supportive peer to activate the dancing dog switch toy. Sam needed prompts to wait for his turn. Sam looked at the "surprise" symbol on the visual timetable. He tried to take it off, and put story-time back in its usual place. I said "surprise – home" and showed him the "surprise" symbol and the "home" symbol to show Sam he is going home early today. We put these on the visual timetable and Sam left them there.	**Expected** Aisha offered a cup to her friend when they were feeding babies in the home corner. There was only one cup, so they took turns feeding the baby. Aisha showed concern when a new child was crying when they came into preschool. Aisha kept looking over to the child. I modelled "sad" on Aisha's talker. Aisha said "want mummy". Aisha was happy for me to show a new member of staff how to use Aisha's communication book with partner-assisted scanning. Aisha cooperated whilst I demonstrated, and then let the new adult try it out.

Starting out with AAC

8. Making relationships	Emerging	Expected
Children play cooperatively, taking turns with others. They take account of one another's ideas about how to organise their activity. They show sensitivity to others' needs and feelings, and form positive relationships with adults and other children.	Sam said sorry to a peer by signing "sorry" with hand-under-hand support. Sam was reminded to use "kind hands" with his behaviour visual support. Sam then shared the same space with the other child for 2 minutes. Sam made brief intense eye contact during some relaxing time in the quiet corner. I was copying the sounds he was making, and Sam stopped and looked at me intently, then carried on with the same happy sounds.	Aisha used the magnetic bricks with two peers to build a "castle" (Aisha told me this using her talker). Aisha smiled when one of her peers brought over the knights and horses from the small-world area and made them climb the castle. Aisha then used her talker to say "climb" and "jump" whilst her peers followed these instructions.

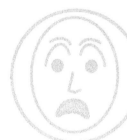

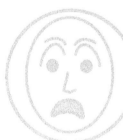

(Continued)

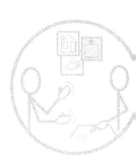

Table 11.7 (Continued)

Area of Learning	Early Learning Goal (ELG)	Sam	Aisha
Literacy	**9. Reading** Children read and understand simple sentences. They use phonic knowledge to decode regular words and read them aloud accurately. They also read some common irregular words. They demonstrate understanding when talking with others about what they have read.	**Emerging** Sam played on the computer with the *Alphablocks* game, bouncing when he played the "watch and sing" animations. Sam recognised the *Thomas the Tank Engine* logo on another child's lunchbox and took this to look closely at it. We matched it to a Thomas train and signed "same". Sam bounced, as if satisfied.	**Expected** Aisha used a *Clicker* grid to match pictures with simple sentences, adapted from *The Tiger Who Came to Tea*, e.g. "the tiger ate all the buns", "the tiger drank all the milk". Aisha used a *Clicker* grid to match CVC words with pictures, e.g. "cot", "cat", "dog", "dig", "sad", "sat". She used the speak function to say them aloud to check they were right.
	10. Writing Children use their phonic knowledge to write words in ways which match their spoken sounds. They also write some irregular common words. They write simple sentences which can be read by themselves and others. Some words are spelt correctly and others are phonetically plausible.	**Emerging** Sam used a stick to make marks in sand. I modelled a circle, and Sam made straight lines. Sam played briefly with the magnetic letters on a board. I spelt "Sam". Sam matched the colours of the letters.	**Expected** Aisha used her onscreen keyboard to write the first two letters in "Aisha", "mummy" and "daddy" and then chose the correct prediction. Aisha used a *Clicker* grid to put words in the correct order to make sentences like "We went to the zoo" and "We saw a big elephant".

Mathematics	**11. Numbers**	**Emerging**	**Expected**
	Children count reliably with numbers from 1 to 20, place them in order and say which number is one more or one less than a given number. Using quantities and objects, they add and subtract two single-digit numbers and count on or back to find the answer. They solve problems, including doubling, halving and sharing.	Sam counts very fast to 10, using a distinctive intonation pattern. Sam enjoys counting songs, like "Five Little Ducks" and joins in with holding the props to go with this song in a small group.	Aisha used the number page on her talker to tell me which number was one more or one less than the number from 1 to 20 that I gave her. Aisha used the number line on her desk to count on two numbers. Aisha used Numicon pieces to show which was half the piece I was holding.
	12. Shape, space and measures	**Emerging**	**Expected**
	Children use everyday language to talk about size, weight, capacity, position, distance, time and money to compare quantities and objects and to solve problems. They recognise, create and describe patterns. They explore characteristics of everyday objects and shapes and use mathematical language to describe them.	Sam used his TEACCH schedule to complete a sorting-by-size activity and a matching coins activity. Sam matched the sequence of three repeated beads on a thread two more times. Sam posted shapes into boxes labelled "triangle", "circle" and "square". These were of varying sizes and colours.	Aisha used her talker to say whether items were "long" or "short" and her peer put them into the correct box. Aisha used the money page on her talker to match the coins I put in front of her. Aisha used her talker to label the shapes "triangle", "square" and "circle" during small-group time.

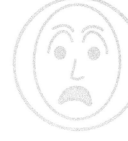

(Continued)

Table 11.7 (Continued)

Area of Learning	Early Learning Goal (ELG)	Sam	Aisha
Understanding the world	**13. People and communities** Children talk about past and present events in their own lives and in the lives of family members. They know that other children don't always enjoy the same things, and are sensitive to this. They know about similarities and differences between themselves and others, and among families, communities and traditions.	**Emerging** Sam brought in a photo of his new baby brother. We made a book about what babies do. Sam shared out the mini packets of sweets he had brought from home for his birthday. With support, he was able to also give his favourite sweets away.	**Expected** Aisha brought in her mum's sari to show the other children. We made Indian sweets and played some bhangra music, which Aisha activated with a switch. Aisha could use her talker to say three things that were the same about her and a peer and three things that were different. She commented on what they like to play with and what they look like.

	Emerging	Expected
14. The world Children know about similarities and differences in relation to places, objects, materials and living things. They talk about the features of their own immediate environment and how environments might vary from one another. They make observations of animals and plants and explain why some things occur and talk about changes.	Sam used the large magnets to pick up smaller objects and put them into a box. Sam looked at a worm found when digging in the raised bed. He poked it with the trowel and jumped when it wiggled. Sam put objects into the water tray in our "floating" experiment. He tried to push them down, and seemed to be experimenting with how much pressure he could exert.	Aisha held a chameleon on our class trip to the reptile park. She used her talker to say it was "shiny" and "dry". When I asked what other animals were like that, Aisha said "snake". Aisha noticed that the soil was dry in the raised bed, and said "need water" using her talker. She had hand-under-hand support to water it with a small watering can.
15. Technology Children recognise that a range of technology is used in places such as homes and schools. They select and use technology for particular purposes.	Sam uses the computer in class for numbers games. He needs support in using it for other applications, and uses a timer to help him stay on-task. Sam is able to shut down games and find the icon for his favourite number game.	Aisha is able to use her talker proficiently in class. Aisha also uses *Clicker* for her written recording. Aisha uses switches to activate the music for assemblies.

(Continued)

Table 11.7 (Continued)

Area of Learning	Early Learning Goal (ELG)	Sam	Aisha
Expressive arts and design	**16. Exploring and using media and materials** Children sing songs, make music and dance, and experiment with ways of changing them. They safely use and explore a variety of materials, tools and techniques, experimenting with colour, design, texture, form and function.	**Emerging** Sam now loves "Wheels on the Bus" and indicates which action he wants next with a supportive adult. He likes to stick with the same order. Sam enjoyed tearing paper and putting it into a big bowl to make papier mâché. Sam used different colour brushes on the interactive whiteboard to make a picture.	**Expected** Aisha used her talker to give alternative farm animals for "Old Macdonald". She chose "dragon" and "unicorn" from the characters page of her talker! Aisha used her talker to give her partner instructions for how to decorate an Easter egg. This included sticking on sequins and feathers.
	17. Being imaginative Children use what they have learnt about media and materials in original ways, thinking about uses and purposes. They represent their own ideas, thoughts and feelings through design and technology, art, music, dance, role play and stories.	**Emerging** Sam built a very tall tower from wooden blocks, climbing on a chair to add blocks to the top. Sam engages in craft materials for 2 minutes. His favourite activity is tearing materials, but does not yet like sticking. Sam is able to engage playing people games, sharing a book and singing songs on a one-to-one basis.	**Expected** Aisha took photos using her talker, and then used these in *Clicker* to make a photo book about our school. She chose the colours and borders of the pages using *Clicker*. Aisha contributed to and recited our class poem in assembly. She used figurative language, comparing a cloud to "a soft pillow".

Home and in the Early Years Setting: The AAC Toolkit

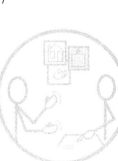

- Provide the same play opportunities with adapted toys.

- Provide regular opportunities to establish cause and effect, e.g. switch toys.

- Provide a communication-friendly environment.

- Provide Aided Language Stimulation throughout the day.

- Encourage multi-modal communication.

- Provide some form of low-tech AAC, including a basic communication chart, an alphabet chart and a number chart.

- Consider positioning, access and mounting.

- Read books every day, commenting, asking and answering questions using AAC.

- Work closely with the Hub and/or Spoke AAC Service to develop low-, light- and high-tech AAC solutions.

- Provide support for the whole family in using AAC.

Notes

1 This relates to the "Enabling Environments" component in the *Statutory Framework for the Early Years Foundation Stage* (2014), found at www.gov.uk.
2 This relates to the "Positive Relationships" component in the *Statutory Framework for the Early Years Foundation Stage* (2014), found at www.gov.uk.
3 http://inclusive.org.uk have a good range of low-tech devices, starting from £5 for *Talking Buttons* and £7 for *Go Talk Buttons, Recordable Thought Clouds* and *Recordable Speech Bubbles*.
4 See http://liberator.co.uk for *Glow Construction Pack* and other light-up products.
5 Latham, C. (2004) *Developing and Using a Communication Book.* Oxford: ACE Centre Advisory Trust.
6 See also *The Key Features of a Communication-Friendly Classroom* on the http://communicationtrust.org.uk website.
7 I would tend not to have a symbol for "good listening" because listening is a bit abstract for young children. It is very difficult for a child to see someone listening. They can see "good looking" and "good sitting" and can copy these more easily. If they are doing these two, they are more likely to be listening anyway.

8 Adapted from Jane Korsten, AAC Specialist. See http://everymovecounts.net/theauthors.

9 Kent-Walsh, J., Hasham, Z. and Stewart, J. (2004) *Instructing Parents to Support Children During Storybook Reading*. Paper presented at the annual convention of the American Speech-Language-Hearing Association, Philadelphia, PA; Binger, C., Kent-Walsh, J., Berens, J., Del Campo, S. and Rivera, D. (2008) Teaching Latino parents to support the multi-symbol message productions of their children who require AAC. *Augmentative and Alternative Communication*, 24, 323–338.

10 Blake, Q. (2012) *Quentin Blake's ABC*. Red Fox.

11 Hand-under-hand is preferred to hand-over-hand because it is more respectful and less controlling for a child with visual impairment, and it means that a child with sensory issues is not forced to touch something (the partner touches it).

12 See Chapter 15 for an overview of AAC Competence, which uses Janice Light's Four Areas of AAC Competencies (Social, Linguistic, Operational, Strategic) as the framework. See Light, J. (1989) Towards a definition of communicative competence for individuals using augmentative and alternative communication systems. *Augmentative and Alternative Communication*, 5, 137–144.

13 As used in Von Tetzchner, S. and Grove, N. (2003) *Augmentative and Alternative Communication: Developmental Issues*. London: Whurr. I have added the dashes to separate symbols.

14 Pugh, D. (2016) *Family perspectives on Augmentative and Alternative Communication*. Presentation given at Communication Matters Conference, Leeds.

15 Ibid.

16 http://communicationmatters.org.uk.

17 http://1voice.info.

18 http://acecentre.org.uk.

19 Contact Kent and Medway Communication and Assistive Technology (CAT) Service for more information.

20 I am indebted to our Kent and Medway CAT Therapy Assistant Practitioners, Clare Ottaway, Amy Williams, Tina Harrison and Sarah Ayres for allowing me to share these session plans.

21 See www.gov.uk. *Early Years Foundation Stage Profile 2016 Handbook*. The Foundation Stage continues to the end of Reception Year at school, but I have included the profile it in this chapter, because evidence will start to be gathered towards the EYFSP in preschool.

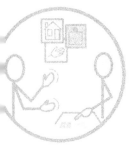

Chapter 12

A new adventure

Starting school

Starting school is momentous for any child and their family. There are likely to be mixed feelings of excitement and trepidation all round.

This chapter is written for all types of school, whether it is a mainstream provision or a special provision. The Code of Practice 2014 states that "the UK Government is committed to inclusive education of disabled children and young people and the progressive removal of barriers to learning and participation in mainstream education".[1] Furthermore, "where a child or young person has SEN but does not have an EHC plan they must be educated in a mainstream setting".[2] Children with Special Educational Needs and Disabilities should be included in "all the opportunities available to other children and young people so that they can achieve well".[3] The Code of Practice goes on to state: "alongside the general presumption of mainstream education, parents of children with an EHC plan and young people with such a plan have the right to seek a place at a special school".[4]

Regardless of whether an AAC user is attending a mainstream or special school, the recommendations in this chapter apply.

The individual AAC user may follow a modified curriculum. There may be a number of therapeutic interventions. It is best practice to integrate this into the classroom where possible. If therapists work within the classroom, they can model strategies for the teaching staff, and they can fine-tune the AAC system to meet the current needs of the child. Opportunities should be available for teaching and therapy staff to plan, do and review[5] together.

The Foundation Stage will continue for another year, but there will be more structured learning in Reception class. The National Curriculum will then begin.

Visual structure for all

All children benefit from visual support. In fact, all adults benefit from visual supports. We use various forms of visual support to organise our thoughts and to support communication. We are more likely to use visual supports when we can't use verbal communication, when we need to process a large amount of information,

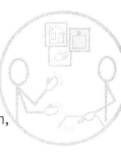

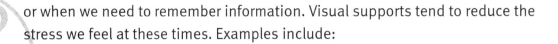

or when we need to remember information. Visual supports tend to reduce the stress we feel at these times. Examples include:

- We follow road signs when we are overseas

- We use icons on our phones and computers

- We put sticky notes around the house

- We write lists

- We write on our hands

- We set reminders on our phones

- We write in diaries or on calendars

- We consult timetables, maps and user guides

- We select from menus

- We follow recipes

- We follow diagrams to build flat-pack furniture

- We red-flag important emails.

Children with processing, memory, or motor planning or behaviour difficulties tend to benefit from visual supports the most. Visual supports save the teacher time in explaining information repeatedly. A quick point to a visual support may be enough to get a child back on track and working independently.

Visual supports that are most useful for AAC users are:

- A low-tech alphabet (preferably with QWERTY layout) on the desk they use;

- A number chart appropriate to their stage of learning;

- A basic communication chart as a backup if their high-tech AAC device is unavailable.

AAC in the classroom

There is no doubt that having a student in the class who uses AAC requires extra skills from the teaching staff. Some basic awareness training from the Hub or Spoke AAC Service is recommended. This might include classroom management strategies such as:

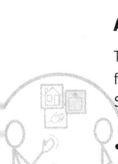

- Thinking about where to position the AAC user and their AAC resources. Some children will need space for their wheelchair or specialist seating, their AAC

device or book, access and mounting. Some children will need to be positioned optimally for their visual or hearing impairment. Some may need modifications to the environment for their sensory processing.

- Managing the set-up of equipment at the start of every lesson. It is recommended that there is a clear routine in place. Every member of the teaching staff knows who is responsible for taking equipment out of the student's bag and positioning it correctly.

- Similarly, making sure that every member of teaching staff has some basic training on how to turn the device on and off, how to change basic settings like volume, how to calibrate for eye-gaze or set up switch-scanning, and how to toggle between communication and curriculum software.

- Taking time to get to know the child's AAC system. It is important for staff confidence that they get to know how vocabulary is organised, how to combine core and fringe vocabulary, how to access an alphabet chart or onscreen keyboard with prediction, how to go back the home screen and how to repeat or delete messages.

- Making use of Teaching Assistant time to prepare AAC resources for the topic (see topic vocabulary charts below), to program relevant vocabulary on the high-tech AAC device, or to make a computer activity on *Boardmaker* or *Clicker*.

- Some activities that are suitable for the AAC user might be useful for the whole class. Interactive whiteboards offer the whole class access to curriculum software. This avoids singling out the AAC user, and in fact can give them the opportunity to be the expert among their peers.

- Leaving enough time for the AAC user to answer class questions. This is a really key management strategy. It is suggested that the teacher ask open questions (wh- questions) unless they need to clarify something with the AAC user. The teacher might address this question to the whole group, or to the AAC user directly. They might then take answers from other classmates, but it is important that they come back to the AAC user to enable them to give their answer to the whole group. There will be times when another child has already answered the question, but the teacher should acknowledge the AAC user's contribution. Another recommended way of managing this is to get other students to write down their answer without shouting out. The AAC user is then asked for their response first.

- In a maths or literacy lesson, the other students may have 10 or 20 short questions to answer in their independent work. Because it takes an AAC user longer to answer each question, they may only have to complete five or 10 questions. So long as they have shown that they understand how to solve this

type of problem (e.g. subtraction), or adding full-stops and capitals, they do not have to laboriously work through every question.

- Managing time to play with the device, and time to focus on work. Parents of AAC users report the importance of their child being able to play on their device, to find out what it can do, to experiment with unfamiliar vocabulary, and to pretend and imagine. It is ideal if there is time built into the school day when an AAC user can use their device playfully, perhaps with peers at break-times. At other times, the AAC user may need prompts to focus on the learning task, and like all other children, will have to learn to regulate the use of their voice appropriately. Visual supports giving a short, positive message (e.g. "listen") can often be most effective here.

Conversation partner training

Basic conversation partner training might be offered to all members of the teaching team. At the least, a staff meeting might be dedicated to teaching the following 10 Top Tips:

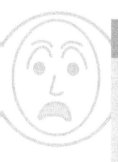

10 Top Tips for New Communication Partners

- Make eye contact, and interact at eye level if possible.

- Introduce yourself.

- Talk directly to the AAC user.

- Check with the AAC user how they indicate "yes" and "no".

- Ask the AAC user to demonstrate how they use their AAC.

- Give the AAC user plenty of time. It's OK to be silent whilst they are using their AAC.

- Don't finish the AAC user's message unless they give you permission.

- Don't ask too many yes/no questions. Ask open questions, or offer comments, and wait for the AAC user to do the same.

- Pay close attention to the AAC user's facial expressions and body language, in case there is misunderstanding. Check you have understood the message correctly.

- Be honest if you don't understand. Ask the AAC user if they can say it in a different way. Seek assistance from a familiar partner if the AAC user gives permission.

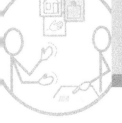

Continued language learning

Typically developing children will be competent language users by school entry but will continue to acquire more sophisticated vocabulary and syntax alongside their literacy learning. There is an interplay between spoken and written language. At first spoken language supports the acquisition of literacy, but then literacy starts to support more sophisticated academic language.

Some children may be at an early stage of language learning, and therefore will need differentiated language input. Aided Language Stimulation should continue, to ensure the level of input attuned to the child (see Chapter 9).

Following are ideas to support continued language-learning across the domains of vocabulary and semantics, grammar and syntax and pragmatics and social skills. AAC learning is incorporated into these ideas. I will then move on to literacy in the following section.

AAC activities to support vocabulary and semantics

Word learning

It is helpful for the teacher to identify key vocabulary in their curriculum planning. At the start of the topic, the teaching staff can check a child's understanding of this key vocabulary. If any words are not yet understood, there may be pre-teaching of vocabulary. In some school settings, many of the children will benefit from this pre-teaching of vocabulary, and so these activities might be for the whole class. To be most effective, vocabulary teaching should incorporate the following[6]:

- *Multisensory, meaningful learning of concepts.* For example, if the concept is "long", then a multisensory, meaningful activity might be for a group of students to compare items that are long and short (e.g. scarves, strings of beads, train tracks, lengths of string, ribbon or wool). They might be encouraged to tie these together to see how far the long length will stretch (e.g. across the playground). Aim for activities to be memorable.

- *The semantic, syntactic and phonological aspects of the new word.* Children might be encouraged to explore these using a visual support. Semantic associations might include "where is it found?" "what is it used for?" "what does it look/sound/feel like?" Syntactic information includes "is it a noun, verb or adjective?" and "can you put it into a sentence?" Phonological components include "how many syllables?" "what does it rhyme with?" "what sound does it start with?" The class might agree and recite a definition of the word, which might be programmed into a light-tech device. Phrases for talking

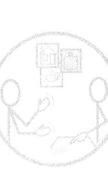

about words are included in the table at the end of the chapter, with vocabulary for English. A really useful resource is a spinner[7] or a dice[8] with six questions about a word, which can be used every time a new word is taught.

- *A way of easily referring back to the new concept.* There might be a "word wall" or a "word box" of new concepts. These can be reviewed regularly. There might be a book of new words, accompanied by photos of the multisensory, meaningful learning activity that was used to teach it. A video of new concepts may even be made, to be shown at regular intervals through the school year.

- *New vocabulary should be added to the child's AAC system.* This might include a low-tech topic vocabulary chart, to be used in all lessons related to this topic. Alternatively it might be added to a child's high-tech VOCA, under the subject or topic category.

- *There should be variety of ways to use the new concept.* The new concept should be used straight away in a variety of structured learning tasks. This might include a low-tech symbolised worksheet or mind-map made with *SymWriter*,[9] *InPrint 3*,[10] *Boardmaker*[11] or *MatrixMaker*.[12] It might include a *Clicker*,[13] *SwitchIt! Maker*[14] or *ChooseIt! Maker*[15] computer activity. It might include using it in a class poem or rap (shown to be useful in recalling new words), in a call-and-response narrative[16] or in a play-script[17] (to help with the functional and social use of the word).

- *Children might be encouraged to rate their knowledge of new vocabulary.* They might include sorting new words into categories of "I understand and use this word", "I know a bit about it, but can't use it yet" and "I don't know this word yet".

Word games

These can be used as filler activities for times in the day when children are waiting for something else to happen, such as lunch and home-time. They are a way of consolidating semantic knowledge. Ideas for word games using AAC include:

- *"I went shopping and I bought. . ."* Each child adds an item to the list. You can vary it, making the category as broad or narrow as you feel is appropriate, for example, "I went on holiday and I took . . .", "I went for a walk to the beach and saw . . ." You can encourage the children to be playful and imaginative, particularly if you know that their categorisation skills are already good.

- *"How many things can you think of that . . ."* Use a wide variety of semantic or phonological associations here. For example "have wheels/legs/a handle/a key"; "can be pushed/pressed/squashed/stretched"; "are soft/cold/wet/tall"; "rhyme with bee", "start with d".

- *"What's in my bag?"* Collect unusual and interesting objects for this. The children have to ask questions to deduce what the object is. For example, "what shape is it?" "who uses it?" "where do we find it?" Encourage the AAC user to use a visual support or their questions page on their AAC system. You might use a spinner[18] or large dice[19] with symbolised "what", "who", "where", "when", "why", and "how" questions.

- *Word association game.* This can be really good fun with children with a reasonable vocabulary. The starting player says a word (or may choose a word from a list or board) and the second person has to think of a related word. An AAC device might come in handy to support other children when they can't think of anything, so that the AAC user has the experience of coming to the rescue for their peers.

- *Shared story-building.* Using a story-frame, with sentence-starters like "Once upon a time there was a . . ." "who went to the . . ." "and found an amazing . . ." "They had a terrible accident with a . . ." "and turned into a . . ." "they felt very . . ." These sentence-starters could be displayed on a spinner or large dice.

AAC activities to support grammar and syntax

Learning specific sentence structures

AAC users make use of more single-word utterances and telegraphic phrases than their typically developing peers.[20] This may be because information can be conveyed more efficiently in a short message. This is provided that there are attuned communication partners who can interpret the message, using non-verbal clues and inference, and who allow the AAC user to correct a misinterpretation. Children using AAC are often assumed to be making requests when they use single symbols, when in fact they may be using other communicative functions, like asking a question, giving information about a present, past or future event, making a joke, and so on.

Children need a critical mass of vocabulary on their AAC system before they can start to combine symbols.[21] They need multiple exposures to a new sentence structure, and multiple opportunities to combine words. It is OK for AAC users to use single symbols to convey urgent and routine information. However, we also want to give them the skills to combine symbols in creative ways to make a range of sentence structures, conveying a range of communicative functions. These are some of the ways we might do this:

- *Aided Language Stimulation,*[22] whereby we model phrases to accompany everything the child is doing, and we add one or two words to what the child

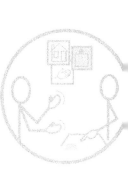

has said. We do this both with their AAC system, and verbally. If they have good understanding of spoken language, then we use full sentences with correct grammar. We model one step ahead of their current expressive AAC, so if they are using single symbols, we model combining two symbols. We might say "she's throwing the ball", as we simultaneously combine the symbols "throw" and "ball". I tend to advise that adults use correct spoken English, and model key words with symbols.

- *Targeted teaching of word combinations*. Pictures, books and video can be used to support teaching of early word combinations, as long as these are accessible. *Colorcards*[23] and other high-quality photo resources are available, which have minimal background distraction, allowing the child to focus on the figures or objects in the foreground. Early word combinations include person + action (e.g. "boy eating"), action + object (e.g. "throwing ball"), person + object (e.g. "dog's ball"), object + position (e.g. "ball in"), object + attribute (e.g. "big ball"). Give the child lots and lots of exposure to the targeted structure before you expect them to use it in a structured learning situation (input before output).

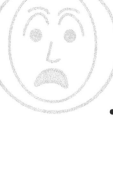

- *Whole-class teaching* of the new sentence structure. Refer to *The National Curriculum*,[24] which includes the use of plural "-s", joining sentences using "and" (Year 1), and using the present tense and past tense (Year 2). These can be demonstrated using *Clicker* grids on an interactive whiteboard, or picture resources like *Colorcards Sequences: Verb Tenses*.[25]

- *Individual practice*, whereby the child takes turns with a communication partner to describe pictures, using their AAC and the targeted sentence structure. Symbolised worksheets might be made using software like *InPrint 3*. Curriculum software like *Clicker* or *ChooseIt! Maker* might be used, whereby the child matches a sentence to a picture, or constructs a sentence using the new sentence structure.

- *Colourful Semantics*[26] is a language intervention that is often used to help sentence-building. There are colour-coded rules depending on whether the word in the sentence is a noun, verb, adjective and so on. This can be useful for some children, but I would not recommend implementing the system across the school for all AAC resources, as this is extremely time-consuming and high-tech AAC vocabulary packages often use their own colour themes.

- *A class book*, made by the students, with photos accompanied by the targeted sentence structure. The book might be added to over the year, with new sentence structures being added. Alternatively this could take the form of a PowerPoint or Adobe presentation.

- *A shared composition and performance.* The sentence structure could be used in a class poem, rap, playscript or story, with the AAC user contributing a line.

General games for grammar

Just like the word games in the previous section, these can be used as quick fillers or as planned activities.

- *Simon Says* can be adapted for a variety of new sentences. For example, if the sentence structure is to learn the adverb "then", the instructions might be in two parts, linked with "then": "touch your toes then clap your hands".

- *Barrier games*, where one student can't see what the other student is looking at, but has to recreate it, can be really useful for practicing giving instructions. For example the AAC user might have to say "the girl kicked the ball", or "put the purple hairy elephant on the orange spotty mouse".

- *Giving instructions* to another student to make food, construct a craft project or carry out a science experiment.

- *Interview a class visitor.* This might be prepared in advance. Each child asks a different question. Or you could conduct a survey asking the same question to many different people around the school (good for maths when making charts).

Activities for AAC to support pragmatics and social skills

- *Structured programmes* such as *Talkabout*[27] may be used if AAC users have particular difficulties with social skills.

- *Playscripts*[28] may be used to target particular communicative functions, for example, greetings, asking questions, repairing misunderstandings. The AAC user might have the target lines in their communication book or programmed onto their device.

- *Role play* is a more creative, spontaneous version of playscripts, whereby the AAC user and their peers are given a scenario and a target skill to practice. This might include asking for directions, ordering food in a café, reporting a problem – the possibilities are endless. If a child is struggling to take part in role play, it may be that they need more core vocabulary, sentence-starters or stored phrases on their device.

- *Show and Tell* are sessions, possibly where the AAC user has prepared their news in advance, if they need to do this. There could be structured questions, using a spinner or large dice with the question options.

- *What's Changed?* One person goes out of the room and changes an aspect of their appearance. You might keep a bag of props like wigs, hats, glasses and shoes for this. The AAC user and their peers have to say what has changed. Or you might change the classroom in some way and see if the students can spot the change. For example, there's a skeleton hanging from the cupboard; there are trays of paint on the floor.

- *Disaster!* Set the students a task, but don't give them everything that they need. Remove a piece of a puzzle or the colour crayon that they need. Or to make it more fun, give them something absurd, like a spade in a cookery activity. Hide something surprising in a container, like a rubber chicken (be cautious for students with ASC or sensory sensitivities). This encourages initiation and problem-solving.

- *Favourites*. Have a large dice or spinning wheel with categories, so that each child can say what is their favourite animal, food, place, activity, colour or book. You could change it to the worst. The possibilities are endless.

- *Agony Aunt*. A puppet has a problem that they need the students to help them with. A social scenario like "I have no one to play with in the playground" is given, and children have to think of suggestions to help. They could choose their three favourite solutions at the end.

Literacy

Literacy is the aim for all AAC users. At the ISAAC[29] conference in 2000, David Yoder said:

No student is too anything to be able to read and write.

Some AAC users may not achieve full literacy, but we want to aim for some functional literacy.

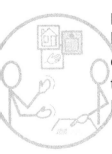

Literacy offers new possibilities for being creative with language. A symbol vocabulary package will only take you so far. But if you can spell even just the first two letters in a word, word prediction software will provide you with an array of words that may not be on your vocabulary package. In many communication packages, these word predictions are symbolised, so that the user does not need to be able to read them already. We should be aiming for all AAC users to have a mix of symbols and an onscreen keyboard with prediction. Some children will progress to a text-only package, with stored quick phrases and sentence-starters, and a keyboard for novel utterances.

AAC users should be given the same access to independent reading for learning and leisure as their non-disabled peers. Literacy opens up a whole world of potential learning. Once a child is literate, they can begin to direct their own learning.

There are several different skills that contribute towards literacy. These will be looked at in turn.

Pre-literacy skills: phonological awareness

These will have started to develop in the Foundation Stage. They do not involve the printed word, but listening to words. Phonological awareness skills include:

- Syllable-awareness: the ability to clap out the syllables in a word (e.g. "e-le-phant", "ti-ger").

- Rhyme awareness: the ability to *hear* the sameness of the end of words (e.g. "plate, gate, eight").

- The ability to generate nonsense rhymes: "mummy, wummy, fummy".

- First sound awareness: being able to sort words into those that start with two different sounds. This is easier if you start with two very different sounds (e.g. "s" and "b").

- Final sound awareness.

- The ability to segment a consonant-vowel-consonant (CVC) word (e.g. "d-o-g", "c-a-t"). It is important that the adult models the short sound (e.g. "d", not "duh"). If children struggle with this, you might segment a word into onset and rime at first (e.g. d-og, c-at).

- The ability to blend CVC words. The adult says the sounds, and the children blend them.

There is obviously a problem here. AAC users cannot produce the sounds to play with words in this way. One solution to this is to encourage the child to use their "inner voice" (see section on 'Inner Voice'). We can also stimulate children's receptive phonological awareness by drawing attention to the sounds in words, and exposing them again and again to syllable-clapping or tapping, rhyme and alliteration.

The best way to develop receptive phonological awareness is through enjoying rhymes and stories spoken aloud. We want to stimulate a child's interest in the sound of words, so that they are motivated to play around with sounds. My favourite books for playing with sounds in words are listed in Table 12.1. Ideas for

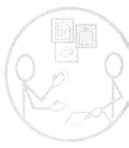

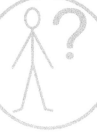

Table 12.1 Books to read

Books for Rhythm, Rhyme and Repetition	
Hairy Maclary From Donaldson's Dairy *Slinky Malinki* Lynley Dodd (Puffin)	These books have nice short lines, making the rhyme stand out. There is also a repeated refrain, which could be programmed on a device, or you could add all of the dog's names, one by one, on a multi-step device. There is brilliant variation in pace, building anticipation and climax with "SCARFACE CLAW the toughest Tom in town". There is brilliant use of sounds with "EEEEEOWWWFFTZ!"
Mr Magnolia *Daisy Artichoke* Quentin Blake (Red Fox)	Once children are familiar with these books, they are brilliant for leaving a gap at the end of the second line, to let children complete it, e.g. "Mr Magnolia has only one boot. He has an old trumpet that goes rooty–" (toot). You might use a multi-step device for this line closure activity.
The Gruffalo *Room on the Broom* Julia Donaldson (Macmillan)	All good for rhythm and rhyme. These are longer books, which are good for children with reasonable attention spans for group reading. The rhyming words could be added to a multi-step device to complete lines.
Fox in Socks Dr Seuss (Harper Collins)	Lots of rhyme, repetition and alliteration. You can just read short sections, if attention starts to wane. You could try making some of the words using the onscreen keyboard of a high-tech device. (You can talk about a silent K in "Knox"!) You could spell new nonsense rhyming words on a device to make new tongue-twisters. You could make ever-longer strings of words, with prepositions in-between, e.g. "bats in hats and cats on mats, cats on bats in hats on mats".
The Book With No Pictures B. J. Novak (Puffin)	No pictures, but really funny text, with lots of nonsense words, to engage and delight children. Program the words "blork" and "bluurf" onto a light-tech device; add the funny phrases onto a multi-step device, or try spelling them on a high-tech device.

using voice-output AAC devices are included. Of course this list is not exhaustive, and teachers will have their own favourites. However I hope there are ideas here to get you started.

Inner voice

We can encourage non-verbal children to use their "inner voice",[30] to say words and letter sounds in their head. The *Non-verbal Reading Approach* (NRA)[31] is a systematic approach, making use of the inner voice to teach children to read CVC words, and then longer words. There is a teaching script to take children through the following sequence for each word:

1   "In your head, say *cat*". (as the teacher holds up the written word)

2   "In your head, say c. Say a. Say t".

3   "In your head, say the sounds altogether. Don't stop between the sounds".

4   "In your head, say the sounds fast".

Once the student has undertaken instruction, they can then be assessed by asking "which one says *cat*?" whilst offering four options. Within the array of four options will be:

1   The target CVC word (e.g. "cat").

2   A word with a different vowel in the middle (e.g. "cot").

3   A word with a different consonant at the end (e.g. "cab").

4   A CVC word with completely different letters (e.g. "bed").

This systematic method of assessing allows the teacher to track the error pattern, and target their teaching accordingly. In the sample assessment, the child could point to the chosen word, or could indicate "yes" as the teacher points to each option.

Literacy and the national curriculum

Synthetic phonics vs. analytic phonics

It is currently recommended that all children are taught *synthetic* phonics, with a heavy reliance on sounding out when reading words. The literature suggests that this is also appropriate for AAC users.[32] However, there is anecdotal evidence within the AAC field that analytic phonics, which emphasises onset and rhyme and building word families (e.g. c-ake, b-ake, m-ake, sn-ake), and thus making more use of visual processing, may be more effective for non-verbal students.

Sight words

As many high-frequency words in English do not conform to phonics rules, these words must be learnt as whole units. Examples include "the", "said" and "two". There is anecdotal evidence to suggest that some non-verbal students learn to read through this method, bypassing phonics altogether, effectively treating all words as if they were sight words. For AAC users, visual processing is often a strength, as they have already had to learn to differentiate many symbols in their AAC system.

It is important not to generalise with AAC users. Each individual will have their unique way of learning to read. The challenge is to find the right strategies and resources for the individual, rather than being evangelical about one particular reading programme. Communication Matters is currently setting up a working party to examine further the most appropriate teaching methods for AAC users, with findings to be shared on their website.

Phonics programmes

There are many different phonics programmes. The National Curriculum allows each school to choose which programme to teach, but it should include the following elements:

- Short, daily sessions to teach all the major grapheme/phoneme correspondences;

- Demonstrating how phonemes are blended and segmented to make CVC[33] words;

- Teaching high-frequency words (sight words) that do not conform to phonics rules;

- Access to texts that are entirely decodable by phonemic strategies.

Examples of synthetic phonics programmes include *Read Write Inc.*,[34] *Letters and Sounds*,[35] *Sounds Write*[36] and *Reading Eggs*.[37] *Phonics for All*[38] is a programme developed specifically for AAC users, incorporating all of the preceding elements, but with analytic phonics too. The programme is computer-based, with a variety of alternative access options, including switch-scanning. The programme encourages the development of an "inner voice" to sound out words internally where speech is not possible. The resource can be used by individuals and groups. It includes a range of activities and progress can be tracked. *The Non-verbal Reading Approach*[39] also makes use of synthetic phonics and is designed with AAC users in mind. This could be combined with any of the mainstream synthetic phonics programmes just listed.

Synthetic phonics programmes can be made accessible to AAC users by incorporating the following:

- Have access to the accompanying software or apps for the phonics programme you are teaching, if they are accessible.

- *ChooseIt! Maker: Literacy* app[40] and related curriculum software packages are all switch-accessible. They comprise a wealth of games in graded steps, covering all of the requirements of a National Curriculum phonics programme.

- Make an alphabet book or a book of targeted phonemes, where each page has one letter, along with corresponding pictures. You could include the symbols the child has in their AAC system.

- Encourage children to also say phonemes in their head, using their "inner voice".[41] All the children in the class might be encouraged to say the phoneme three times aloud, and three times in their head. The AAC user may use their inner voice when they are reading phonemes, words, and later text. The inner voice allows us to read silently, which AAC users have to do.

- Programme two single-message devices with two different letter sounds, labelled with the grapheme. Present the group with words, symbols or pictures of words that start either one of those sounds. Encourage the AAC user to help to decide which sound they start with.

- Programme a multiple-overlay device with a page of phonemes that are being targeted, so that the AAC user can take part in group activities.

- Use *Talking Photo Books*[42] or *Talking Speech Bubbles*[43] programmed with the targeted letter name or sound, with teaching resources showing words beginning with the target sound.

- Use the child's onscreen keyboard for blending CVC words. These onscreen keyboards do not say letter sounds, but letter names. If letter sounds are preferred, you may choose to record these onto the device. However, the child will need to learn letter names too, so there is an argument for leaving them as they are.

- Have a low-tech alphabet chart available on AAC user's desk. This might be a screenshot of their high-tech onscreen keyboard, if the size and colour

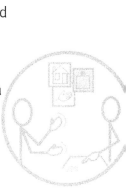

contrasts are appropriate. The alphabet chart may be part of a low-tech communication chart that is always available. A number chart is also useful to include in this. Lowercase letters are preferred when teaching early literacy.

- Draw attention to the core words in the child's AAC system. These are often high-frequency sight-words that can be learnt as whole words. You can prioritise the core words the child has on their home screen for their reading words first. Add the other high-frequency sight-words to the child's AAC system as you introduce them to the class.

- If the AAC user is successfully reading and using some of these high-frequency sight words, it may be decided to remove the symbol and have the text only for these words in their AAC system.

Sentence-level work

We have looked at phonics and sight words, which are strategies for reading and writing at a word level. Now we will consider reading and writing at the sentence level.

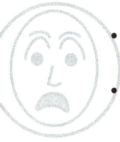

- Use the *Chooselt! Literacy* app or *Clicker* software to start to read sentences. *Clicker* books can be useful for this. These are included in *Clicker 7*.

- Use curriculum software, like *Clicker* "sentence sets" and "connect sets" to build sentences. The software will model the sentence to be made, and will speak the sentence that the child has made, to provide instant feedback. Here are some examples of sentence-building tasks, in order of difficulty:

  1 Arranging words in a sentence. Start with three or four words. Only these three or four words are available, but the child has to put them in the right order.

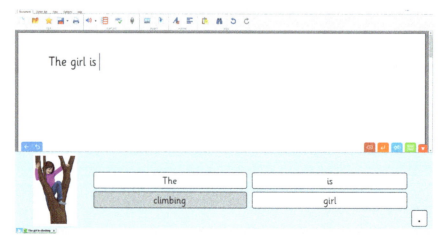

Figure 12.1 The girl is

2 Arranging words in a sentence, but with different options for one of the words.

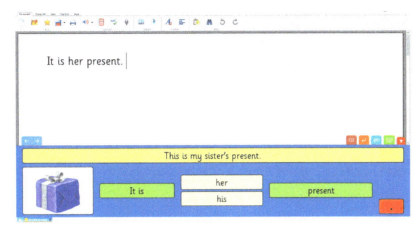

Figure 12.2 It is her present

3 Making a sentence with multiple options for more than one word in the sentence.

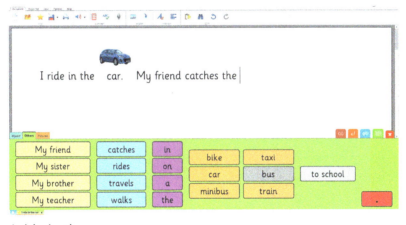

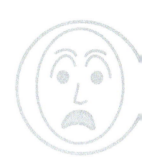

Figure 12.3 I ride in the car

4 Using "word banks". These can be extensive collections of vocabulary around a given topic. Words may be organised by topic, or alphabetically, by using tabs. The child can then produce pieces of written work in a variety of formats.

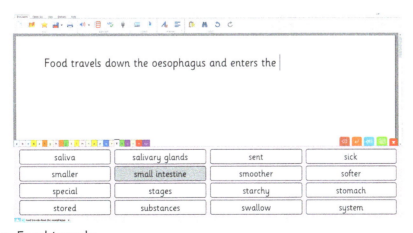

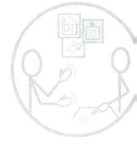

Figure 12.4 Food travels

5 Using "spelling prediction" to increase independent writing. If prediction is turned on, then when a child starts to type a word, five or more alternatives will appear in a pop-up. The child can then select the word they want. They can listen to the words if they need to. Spelling prediction can be combined with word banks or used on its own. The spelling prediction can be personalised for a child's commonly misspelt words. Children are often motivated to use more complex vocabulary and sentences by using prediction.

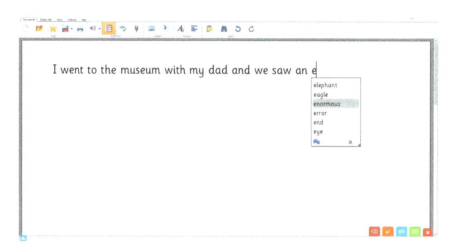

Figure 12.5 I went to the museum

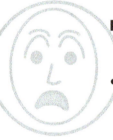

- Low-tech alternatives can be used for the first three stages. However, make sure that such activities are not hindered by a child having to cut and stick resources. Children are often slowed down by the visual processing, fine motor and motor-planning demands, leaving very little capacity for the language demands of the task. Computer-based sentence-construction tasks often require less physical effort, sensory processing and motor-planning. A child's success will often lead to greater motivation and engagement for writing activities.

Reading comprehension

It is vital that a child reads for meaning. There a few different things that we can do to support reading comprehension:

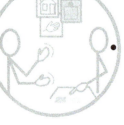

- Read picture books without any words. Early reading involves a lot of guesswork, using the picture for clues. Therefore we want the AAC user to get used to reading the pictures too! *Oxford Reading Tree*[44] produce books with no words.

- Read books without pictures, and encourage the child to make pictures in their head. Start off with simple narratives you have made up, like "once there was a dragon. Can you see the dragon? He's green and scaly and huge, and he breathes fire!" Making pictures in our head as we read, or *visualising*, helps with reading comprehension.[45]

- Read picture books and link the text with the picture. You might want to use a pointer with a light, to highlight text and details of the picture in group reading.

- You can then use pictures from the story in *SwitchIt! Maker*,[46] *Choose It! Maker*[47] or *Clicker*,[48] and encourage the child to match the picture with the text. These can be a group activity on the interactive whiteboard or on a class computer.

- Encourage the child to use their language skills to predict the end of sentences, using what they have learnt from the picture. If you are focusing on a book for a term, then have these words available on a low-tech topic sheet[49] or low-tech device.

- Read the same story several times, building a greater understanding with familiarity.

- Think aloud: add your own thoughts about the story as they occur to you to model this skill. For example, wonder aloud what might happen next or why a character might be doing what they are doing. This shows that reading is an active process, and that we make sense of text as we go along.

- Check back a child's understanding of what has happened every now and again, but don't make it a test. You can summarise or paraphrase the text to support their understanding.

- A good way to monitor understanding of a text is to stop at a given point, and ask the children to write their own ending. The AAC user might do this using their AAC system or curriculum software such as *Clicker*.

- Talk about the meaning of new words and phrases, and any imagery in the text. Model the meaning on the child's AAC system (e.g. for "guava" you might say "green and pink fruit").

- Have extension activities around a book, exploring the themes of the book. For example for *Handa's Surprise*[50] the class could try some of the fruit from the story.

- Consider acting out a story, or use props as you read a story, to make it more memorable and tangible. Again for *Handa's Surprise*, children could pretend to be the various animals.

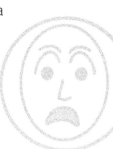

- Don't be tempted to symbolise written text if you are working on reading words. Adding symbols may draw attention away from the written text. The general rule is to use symbol support when you are working on comprehension of language, but don't use it if you are working on reading.[51]

Whole-class reading, guided reading and self-chosen reading

There should be a balance between these. Whole-class reading might include a "big book" or the book pages shown on the interactive whiteboard. The text might be highlighted as the teacher reads it, or specific words might be discussed. Guided reading is where an adult will read the text with a group, but each child will have access to their own copy of the text. Children might take turns to read. The text will be discussed. Self-chosen reading is where a student selects the book they want to read. Sometimes teachers might narrow the choice to books that are linked to a class topic. The teacher might encourage a child to read a different type of text (e.g. non-fiction).

AAC users will have no option but to read silently in their head. Don't be tempted to make them say the words as they read them using their AAC, because this will add too much cognitive load, and will break the flow of their reading. Teaching staff have to have faith that the AAC user is reading along with the others. You can check that they *are* reading in the sentence-level activities. Whole-class reading, guided reading and self-chosen reading should be about immersing the child in the text, getting the overall gist and enjoying the flow of the story.

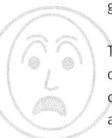

There is no advantage of electronic or audio books at this stage. The preferred option is a responsive communication partner to support book-reading. When a child is already a proficient reader, then electronic resources may come in useful, as they may be more accessible and allow for independent reading.

Tar Heel Readers[52] is an online resource of accessible books on a range of topics. These are text-to-speech enabled, and can be accessed with a range of methods, including switch-scanning. These are mainly non-fiction books and are not organised according to level of difficulty, so they require an experienced teacher to guide the student in making a selection.

Books for All,[53] created by CALL Scotland, is an excellent website offering information and alternative formats of a huge range of mainstream books, including early readers like *Oxford Reading Tree*, children's classics, teen fiction and text books. The website allows teachers and parents to search for titles on a database and request digital copies. The alternative formats include text-to-speech reading and symbolised text.

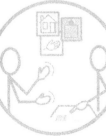

Continue to read aloud to children into secondary school

Children have to learn the specific language of books. The language in books can be different to spoken language. The language of storybooks tends to make more use of repetition, alliteration and rhyme. It tends to take a more stylised form. There are interesting words and phrases that we might not use every day in spoken language. Once we are literate, most of the new words we learn are those we encounter through reading.

We should continue to read aloud to children long after they have learnt to read themselves. We can talk about new words, explain the meaning of long sentences and figurative language. Reading stories helps to foster empathy and emotional understanding of ourselves and others. It offers a much wider experience of the world. I think that the development of imagination is particularly important for children with physical and sensory impairments. We need to tap into this inner resource to stimulate creative expression.

Table 12.2 includes favourite books for firing the imagination, encouraging reasoning and increasing emotional awareness. Of course there are many more books that do this, but this selection is here to give ideas about how AAC can be used.

Table 12.2 Books . . .

Books to Fire the Imagination	
Angelica Sprocket's Pockets *Patrick* Quentin Blake (Red Fox)	Angelica Sprocket has various absurd items in her pockets. Use a child's ACC system to choose other ridiculous items. Play a describing guessing game for the things Angelica has in her pockets, e.g. "we eat it; it's cold; it's sweet" Patrick's violin-playing makes fish fly, changes the colours of leaves and covers cows with stars. Talk about what other magical things might happen, giving some support if needed, e.g. what might happen to flowers? Clouds? Whales?
Would You Rather? John Burningham (Red Fox)	Various absurd options, like "would you rather . . . your house were surrounded by water, snow or jungle?" "a pig tried on your clothes or a hippo slept in your bed?" Brilliant for exploring different pages of vocabulary and combining words to make phrases. Use a child's AAC device to think of more silly options.

(Continued)

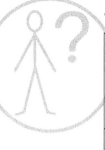

Table 12.2 (Continued)

Tatty Ratty Helen Cooper (Corgi)	Tatty Ratty, a lost toy, goes to various amazing places and has adventures. Use a child's AAC to add other places he might go and things he might do.
I Am Not Sleepy and I Will Not Go To Bed Lauren Child (Orchard Books)	What else might you do so you don't have to go to bed? What scares you at night? What would make these things funny instead? Use the actions, animals and characters pages of the child's AAC system to generate ideas.
Books for Reasoning	
Dr Xargle's Book of Earthlets Jeanne Willis and Tony Ross (Andersen Press)	This is told from the perspective of an alien, teaching alien children about Earth babies. Encourage children to work out what the words refer to, e.g. what are a baby's tentacles with feelers? (arms and hands) What is the hole in their face? Why would they explode? Choose other things on Earth for children to explain to an alien, e.g. dogs, cars, schools.
Princess Smartypants Babette Cole (Puffin)	Good for talking about gender expectations and story conventions. Talk about absurdities in the pictures, e.g. the horse on the sofa, the giant slug in the garden. Why is that funny? Talk about what might happen next in the pictures, asking "how" and "why" questions.
Books for Discussing Difference, Diversity and Friendship	
Elmer the Elephant David McKee (Andersen Press)	Good for talking about difference, and emotions around feeling left out. Talk about how you would decorate yourself on Elmer's special day. What materials would you use? Talk about personality traits that make you or your friends special.

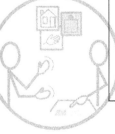

Yuk Kes Gray and Nick Sharratt (Red Fox)	Good for talking about being an individual. Talk about Daisy's and her mum's feelings and how they reach a compromise. Share opinions about Daisy's outfits, or what you might like to wear if you would design your own outfits.
Mr Podd and Mr Piccalilli Penny Dolan and Nick Sharratt	Good for talking about loneliness and friendship. Good for comparing what is the same and what is different about Mr Podd and Mr Piccalilli, their possessions, and the things they do.

Handwriting

Recently a parent presented me with two literacy books showing her daughter's work.

One book contained mainly handwritten pieces of work. The writing was not easy to read. Some letters were well-formed, but others were not. The handwriting looked as though it had been effortful. The vocabulary was basic, as was the sentence construction. The pieces of work were limited to two or three sentences. All the hand-drawn pictures were the same stick figures. There was no evidence of progression over the academic year.

The second book contained examples of the same student's work completed using *Clicker* software. These pieces of work looked professional and interesting, with pictures and photos sometimes accompanying the text. There was interesting and varied vocabulary. There was a range of sentence types, including different connectives and pronouns. Punctuation was often used, with capital letters and full stops. The work was *easy to read*. If the student had wanted to read and enjoy her own work, she could have, and she would have taken pride in the quality of the finished look.

When this student was given access to appropriate curriculum software, she could show what she was really capable of. When she had to laboriously sit and copy words out by hand, most of her cognitive effort went into her fine motor control, visual processing and motor planning. This was a waste of effort, and did not allow her to focus her energies on the creative and rewarding process of writing.

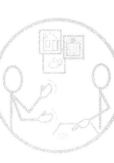

Handwritten news

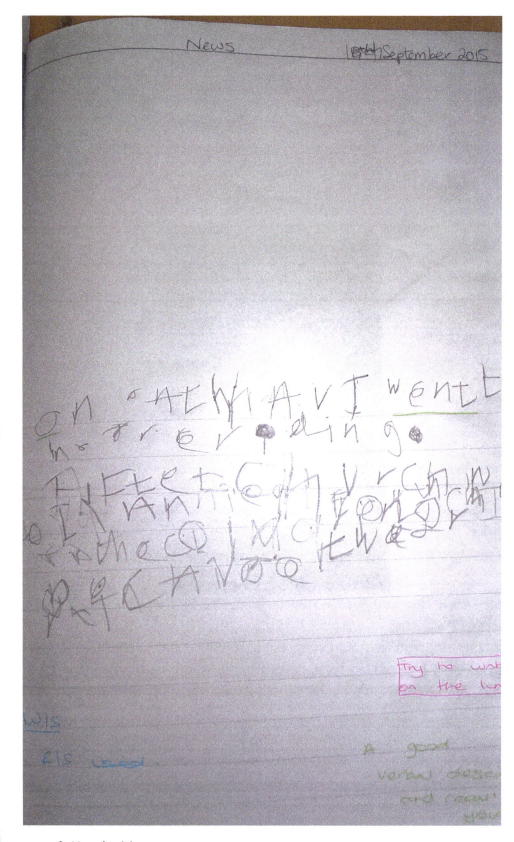

Figure 12.6 Handwriting

Creative writing using *Clicker*

> In a strange, faraway land there lived an old man.
> He lived in a falling down hut in the middle of a forest.
> One dark, still night he was waiting for a bus when he heard a short, low whistle.
> Next there appeared a glidin‍ monster it flew around and around, cackling.
> The old man ran home and locked the door.

Figure 12.7 Clicker

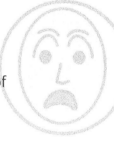

I recognise a need for an AAC user to sign their name. They may need to sometimes write a list or a quick note. Scribes are often used in schools, and this has a place. A scribe is best used in situations where it is not practical to use word processing software, where a quick note to peers or a teacher might contribute to a shared task. But for quality recording of a student's learning, and for creative expression of their ideas, then they have to have access to technology.

The wider curriculum

Topic vocabulary sheets

These are specific visual supports for the topic being covered. Examples are shown in Figures 12.8 and 12.9. Topic vocabulary sheets are used to supplement vocabulary on a child's AAC system. There are some good reasons for not adding this to the AAC system permanently. If the AAC system is low- or light-tech, it might take up too much of the system's capacity, not leaving room for essential core vocabulary and higher-frequency fringe vocabulary. The vocabulary might be very specific to the topic (e.g. if the topic was "Romans" or "Wonders of the World"). It might only be used for a term, and therefore would not be functional in the following term. Even high-tech devices can get clogged up with vocabulary that is not used regularly. There is the danger that if multiple adults add vocabulary, then they might inadvertently duplicate vocabulary that is already on the device. Therefore sometimes, a low-tech topic vocabulary sheet is the answer. This resource may be kept in a file to be used in a later key stage, if it is a recurring curriculum theme.

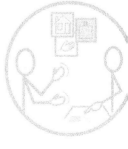

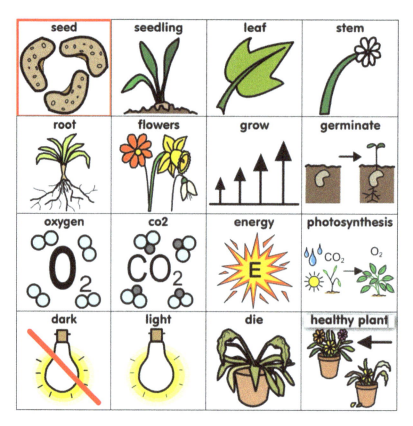

Figure 12.8 Plant growth

Topic vocabulary sheet for "Plant Growth"

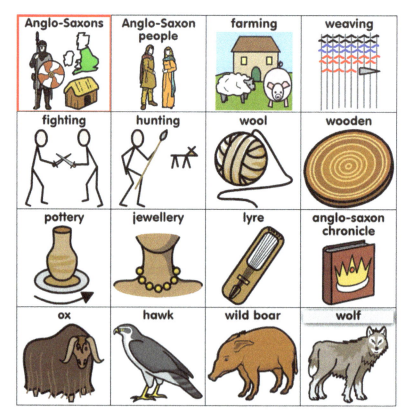

Figure 12.9 Anglo-Saxons

Topic vocabulary sheet for "Anglo-Saxons"

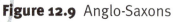

Table 12.3 shows the different subjects in the National Curriculum for Key Stages 1 and 2, and the key vocabulary for each. This is the vocabulary that I consider to be most useful for an AAC system. Other fringe vocabulary may be as important for a particular topic, but might be best on a topic vocabulary sheet. If a child has an extensive vocabulary package (e.g. *Proloquo2Go* or *SymbolTalker B*), then it is useful to have subject folders under the main "school" folder. Lots of this vocabulary will already be in the package, so don't duplicate it: instead you might be able to add links to existing folders. Discuss vocabulary organisation with the child's Speech and Language Therapist to avoid confusion and duplication.

Table 12.3 Software

Subject	Key Concepts
English	*Opinions*: I think that . . . It makes me feel . . . I like it because . . . I don't like it because . . . It reminds me of . . . It makes me think about . . . *Words*: It looks like . . . It sounds like . . . It is like . . . It is the opposite of . . . It rhymes with . . . It begins with . . . These phrases can be used for word learning and word games, but also conversation repair. *Questions*: who, what, where, when, why, how. *Emotions*: happy, sad, angry, frightened, frustrated, disappointed, etc. *Keyboard*: QWERTY, ABC or high-frequency as appropriate; punctuation. Word prediction is recommended. *Books*: cover, spine, page, paragraph, line, sentence, word. *Genres*: story, poem, play, diary, letter, newspaper report, fiction, non-fiction. *Grammar*: core words will already be on the AAC system, and grammar options may be available.
Maths	*Numbers*: 1–10 initially, then 1–20 and then 1–100. *Shapes*: circle, square, triangle, rectangle, hexagon, pentagon. Later, 3D shapes: sphere, cube, cuboid, prisms, symmetry, rotation. *Size*: big, small, full, empty, long, short, tall, heavy, light. *Position*: up, down, top, bottom, in, on, under, left, right.

(*Continued*)

Table 12.3 (Continued)

Subject	Key Concepts
	Calculations: add, subtract, multiply, divide, equals. *Quantity*: Lots, none, more, less, double, half. *Money*: 1p, 2p, 5p, 10p, 50p, £1, £2, £5, £10, £20. Shown in coins and notes. *Fractions*: 1/2, 1/3, 2/3, 1/4, 3/4, 1/5, etc. Best if shown visually. *Comparing*: Be careful about introducing comparatives and superlatives, e.g. bigger, smaller, biggest, smallest. Make sure the basic adjective is secure first, e.g. big and small. Grammar options may be available on the child's high-tech AAC. *Time*: days of the week, months of the year, times of the day. Yesterday, today, tomorrow, last week, next week, last year, next year, before, after, early, later, quick, slow. Measurements: km, m, cm, mm; kg, g; l, ml
Science	**KS1:** *Plants:* plant, tree, leaf, stem, root, flower, petal, stamen, stigma, seed, bulb, trunk, bark, deciduous, evergreen, nutrients, light, water. *Animals*: mammal, bird, fish, reptile, amphibian, insect; carnivore, herbivore; fur, feathers, scales, wings, fins. *Human body*: head, neck, arms, elbows, legs, knees, face, ears, eyes, hair, mouth, teeth, bones, muscle. *Materials*: wood, plastic, glass, metal, water, rock, cardboard. *Describing*: hard/soft; stretchy/stiff; shiny/dull; rough/smooth; bendy/not bendy.
	KS2: *Investigating*: light, sound, force, friction, magnetic, electric, transparent, soluble, conductive. *Human body*: brain, heart, lungs, stomach, intestines, bowel, liver, kidneys, bladder, blood. *States of matter*: solid, liquid, gas, freezing, melting, evaporating, condensing, solution, dissolving. *Space*: Sun, Moon, Earth, Solar System, Mercury, Venus, Earth, Mars, Jupiter, Saturn, Uranus, Neptune, Pluto.

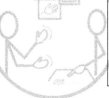

Subject	Key Concepts
Geography	*Places*: UK, England, Wales, Scotland, Northern Ireland. Include major cities of UK; continents and significant countries of the world. *Weather*: sunny, rainy, cloudy, snow, storm, thunder, lightning, fog. *Geographical features*: beach, cliff, coast, forest, hill, mountain, sea, ocean, river, soil, valley. *Man-made features*: city, town, village, factory, farm, house, office, port, harbour and shop (these will be in Places: don't duplicate).
History	King, Queen, Stone age, Bronze age, Iron age, Roman, Viking, Anglo-Saxon, Norman, Tudors, Stuarts, Georgians, Victorians. (And pages already on the device, e.g. *People, Home, Places, Actions, Describing, Opinions, Feelings*)
Art	This will use pages already on the device, e.g. *Art and Craft, Actions, Colours, Shapes, Describing, Opinions, Feelings*.
Music	This will use pages already on the device, e.g. *Music, Actions, Describing, Opinions, Feelings*.
PE	This will use pages already on the device, e.g. *Parts of the Body, Actions*.
Languages	This is controversial. There is a lack of research into AAC users learning an additional spoken language. It will depend upon the cognitive level and educational attainment of the individual, as well as personal choice. I would be inclined to focus on other skills, rather than learn another spoken language at this stage.

Curriculum software

We have already discussed curriculum software including *SwitchIt!*, *ChooseIt!* and *Clicker* for literacy. These resources support the wider National Curriculum too. There is no need to reinvent the wheel: there is a wealth of ready-made resources. *ChooseIt! Ready-Mades* are resources for literacy, maths and science in Key

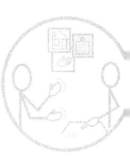

Stages 1 and 2. Similarly, once *Clicker* software or apps have been purchased, a wealth of online resources can be selected.[54] *Splash!*[55] is a piece of software for maths, science and drawing which allows students to set out calculations, and to make use of graphs, charts and geometry activities. *Kidspiration*[56] is another piece of software that can be particularly helpful for learning maths concepts. Many of the resources that are commonly used to make maths meaningful cannot be manipulated by a child with severe physical impairments. *Kidspiration* maths software translates these into computer graphics (e.g. hundreds, tens and ones blocks and fractions tiles), to allow students to solve problems visually. There are a few examples of each of these resources in Figures 12.10 through 12.15.

E Counting sides - 20   Page: 1 of 20   Press Esc to stop   Time: 0m 34s

Which shape has 4 sides?

Figure 12.10 Shapes

ChooseIt! *Maths Activities*

P Symmetry is   Press ESC when you want to stop   Page 4 out of 20

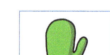

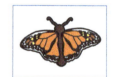

Which shape is symmetrical?

Figure 12.11 Symmetrical

ChooseIt! *Maths Activities*

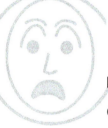

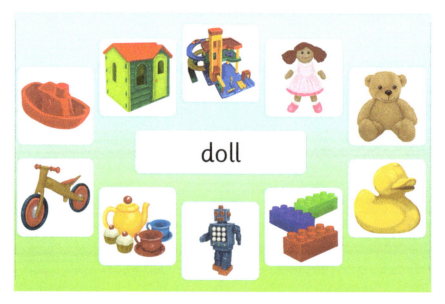

Figure 12.12 Doll

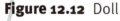
Clicker 7 *set for word-picture matching*

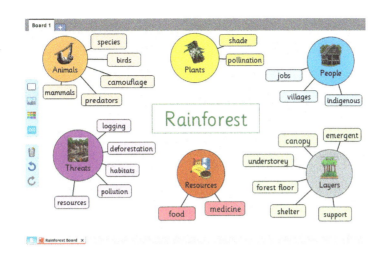

Figure 12.13 Rainforest

Clicker 7 *mind-map*

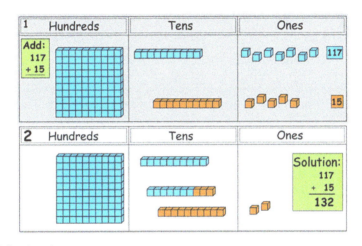

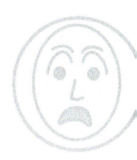

Figure 12.14 Kidspiration

Kidspiration *1000s, 100s, 10s and 1s activity*

These screenshots were taken from Kidspiration(R) 3, a product of Inspiration(R) Software, Inc.

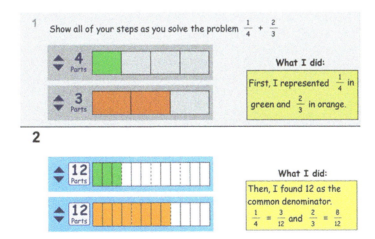

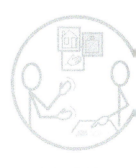

Figure 12.15 Fractions

Kidspiration *fractions activity*

These screenshots were taken from Kidspiration(R) 3, a product of Inspiration(R) Software, Inc.

Go Worksheet Maker[57] is an app that allows you to convert printed worksheets to iPad activities. The teacher can customise how the student completes activities. This may include tapping on multiple-choice answers, dragging and dropping items, drawing a line to connect items, using word banks or the onscreen keyboard.

Social participation

Studies have found that the ability to participate in social recreation is important for the social status and the self-esteem of an individual, and for their ability to develop friendships.[58] There need to be opportunities for friendships to be established, both spontaneously or in a structured way.

For spontaneous friendships to become established, the AAC Team need to build in social competency targets, such as the AAC user being able to introduce themselves, and to say something about the way they communicate. They need to have appropriate vocabulary and phrases for chatting.

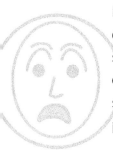

For more structured initiation of new friendships, teaching staff might decide on deliberate groupings of children for learning tasks and leisure pursuits. A supportive (but not intrusive) adult might be on hand to make suggestions in case of communication breakdown. Some schools have successfully operated a buddy system for all new students and playground support systems for bringing together pairs or groups of children to play.

An ethos of inclusion and an interest in and respect for diversity should be fostered in all schools. Parents have an important role to play in fostering social values, and so they should be included in any awareness-raising. This sort of work must take place at a strategic level in school, involving the Senior Management Team, and be part of the school's vision.

Resources are available to educate children about disability; an example is Marion Stanton's book *Can I Tell You About Cerebral Palsy?*[59] Just Different[60] is an organisation that present positive and inspiring workshops about disability and being different for children and young people. The Disability Action Alliance[61] have links to a wealth of teaching resources on their website.

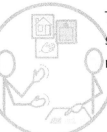

The Equality Act 2010[62] sets out a clear expectation that schools should provide the same range of experiences for children and young people with disabilities as their non-disabled peers. This includes access to learning outside the classroom and

extracurricular clubs. Reasonable adjustments include extra staffing and accessible transport.

Schools have a duty to promote the interests of disabled people and foster good relationships between disabled children and their non-disabled peers. A culture which celebrates diversity and difference should be fostered and promoted between parents of disabled and non-disabled children, as this will increase children's participation out of school too. Opportunities for parents to socialise within school is likely to lead to increased socialisation outside of school. This might include invitations to parties and playdates. These issues require sensitive handling, however, so that the disabled child doesn't feel singled out.

The Local Offer[63] sets out information about extracurricular resources for children and young people. In addition there will be mainstream clubs and groups, for example Brownies and Cubs, Sports, dance and music classes. The Equality Act 2010[64] promotes social participation in such groups, but there has been little research into the take-up of extracurricular activities by children with SEND.

During primary school, social participation is likely to be negotiated via the child's family, teachers and therapy staff. Consideration should be given to social participation when EHCP outcomes are being written and reviewed.[65]

An AAC user's participation in social activities might be promoted in the following ways:

- Parents, siblings and peers model how to use the AAC system with the AAC user in social situations.

- A "Chat" page is included in the child's AAC system to allow them to introduce themselves, give information and ask questions.

- Relevant vocabulary for the child's social activities is included in their AAC system, including phrases for playground games.

- A "News" page is included in the child's AAC system, which allows them to share what they have been doing outside of school.

- Help children to explore their likes and dislikes with their peers, to develop a sense of their identity and what they have in common with other children.

- A buddy system or a supportive friendship circle may be introduced, and carefully monitored.

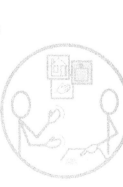

- The AAC user should be consulted about after-school clubs they might like to join.

- Quiet activities can sometimes be most effective and enjoyable as a basis for establishing friendships. Craft, board games and TV have been reported to be a common shared activities enjoyed by AAC users and their peers.[66]

- Positive messages about disability and social participation around the school. For example a focus on the Paralympics, or on high-profile AAC users like Stephen Hawking, Kate Caryer,[67] Toby Hewson[68] and Martin Pistorius.[69]

- Representation of AAC in school newsletters, performances, awards and displays.

Child protection

All children should be given information about types of abuse and how to protect themselves and report concerns. The NSPCC produce materials for schools and services to use to talk to children about abuse, including their "PANTS" guidelines.[70] For a child to access this resource, and to report concerns, they need the following vocabulary on their AAC system:

- Parts of the body and clothing.

- The concept of "private". This might be in "adjectives", and may be linked to "parts of the body".

- The concept of "secret". I would suggest that this is also in "adjectives" and could be linked to "parts of the body".

- Verbs for different types of touch (e.g. "push", "pull") and for different types of talk (e.g. "whisper", "shout").

- Adjectives like "bad" and feelings like "frightened".

Children should be encouraged to think about adults they trust and could talk to about concerns.

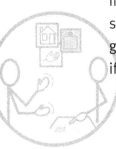

If a disclosure is made, then the adult should always take verbatim notes or screenshots of what a child has said and what the adult said. Local child protection guidelines should be followed, and advice from an AAC Specialist should be sought if a child or young person is to be interviewed.

Primary School: The AAC Toolkit

- Provide appropriate visual supports.

- Provide basic conversation partner training.

- Provide Aided Language Stimulation throughout the day.

- Encourage multi-modal communication.

- Provide low-tech AAC, including a basic communication chart, alphabet chart and number chart.

- Consider positioning, access and mounting.

- Provide high-quality literacy teaching.

- Provide appropriate curriculum software.

- Work closely with the Hub and/or Spoke AAC Service to monitor and adapt light- and high-tech AAC solutions.

- Consider social inclusion across school contexts.

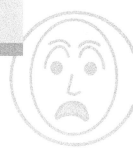

Notes

1 www.gov.uk. *Special Educational Needs and Disability the Code of Practice: 0–25* (2014), p. 25.
2 Ibid.
3 Ibid., p. 26.
4 Ibid., p. 28.
5 Ibid., pp. 101–102.
6 See Parsons, S. and Branagan, A. (2014) *Word Aware: Teaching Vocabulary Across the Day, Across the Curriculum*. Speechmark for more ideas about vocabulary-learning.
7 A low-tech cardboard spinner might be constructed, or you might invest in the *All Turn It Spinner*, which is switch-activated, available from http://inclusive. co.uk. Six different symbols may correspond with the numbers on the spinner.
8 Large dice can be used with a variety of collections of six symbols with the aid of Velcro. There is a light-tech dice called the *Chatterblock* available from http:// inclusive.co.uk, on which you can display symbols and record a corresponding message for each face of the dice.
9 https://widgit.com.
10 Ibid.

11 http://inclusive.co.uk.

12 Ibid.

13 http://cricksoft.com/uk.

14 http://inclusive.co.uk and http://helpkidzlearn.com.

15 http://inclusive.co.uk and http://helpkidzlearn.com.

16 See http://lisntell.co.uk for brilliant ideas about how to use group narratives with children with complex communication needs.

17 See Robertson, S. and Weismer, S. (1996) The influence of peer models on the play scripts of children with specific language impairment. *Journal of Speech, Language and Hearing Research*, 40(1), 49–61.

18 A low-tech cardboard spinner might be constructed, or you might invest in the *All Turn It Spinner*, which is switch-activated, available from http://inclusive.co.uk. Six different symbols may correspond with the numbers on the spinner.

19 Large dice can be used with a variety of collections of six symbols with the aid of Velcro. There is a light-tech dice called the *Chatterblock* available from http://inclusive.co.uk, on which you can display symbols and record a corresponding message for each face of the dice.

20 Blockberger, S. and Sutton, A. (2003) Language experiences and knowledge of children with extremely limited speech. In Light, J., Beukelman, D. and Reichle, J. (eds.), *Communicative Competence for Individuals Who Use AAC: From Research to Effective Practice*. Baltimore: Paul H. Brookes, pp. 72–73.

21 See Chapters 2 and 4.

22 See Chapter 9.

23 http://speechmark.net. Particularly useful are *Colorcards Basic Verbs, Adjectives* and *Prepositions* and *Pocket Colorcards Early Actions* and *Silly Pictures*.

24 www.gov.uk. *National Curriculum in England: English Programmes of Study: Key Stages 1 and 2*.

25 http://speechmark.net.

26 Bryan, A. (1997) Colourful semantics: Thematic role therapy. In S. Chiat, J. Law and J. Marshall (eds.), *Language Disorders in Children and Adults: Psycholinguistic Approaches to Therapy*. Chapter 3.2 London: Whurr. Published online: 15 Apr 2008, doi:10.1002/9780470.

27 Kelly, A. (2016) *Talkabout: A Social Communication Skills Package, 2nd Edition*. Speechmark.

28 See Robertson, S. and Weismer, S. (1996) The influence of peer models on the play scripts of children with specific language impairment. *Journal of Speech, Language and Hearing Research*, 40(1), 49–61.

29 The International Society for Augmentative and Alternative Communication (ISAAC) Conference 2000. DJI-AbleNet Literacy Lecture by David Yoder.

30 From Erikson, K. and Koppenhaver, D. (2007) *Children With Disabilities: Reading and Writing the Four-Blocks Way*. Greensboro, NC: Carson-Dellosa.

31 Coleman-Martin, M., Wolf Keller, K., Cihak, D. and Irvine, K. (2005) Using computer-assisted instruction and the non-verbal reading approach to teach word identification. *Focus on Autism and Other Developmental Disabilities*, 20(2), 80–90.

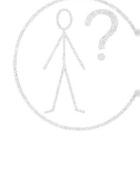

32 Barker, M., Saunders, K. and Brady, N. (2012) Reading Instruction for children who use AAC: Considerations in the pursuit of generalizable results. *Augmentative and Alternative Communication*, 28(3), 160–170.

33 http://consonant-vowel-consonant.

34 http://ruthmiskin.com.

35 http://letters-and-sounds.com.

36 http://sounds-write.co.uk.

37 http://readingeggs.co.uk.

38 Marion Stanton, *Phonics for All* at http://thinksmartbox.com.

39 Heller, K., Fredrick, L., Tumlin, J. and Brineman, D. (2002) Teaching decoding for generalization using the nonverbal reading approach. *Journal of Developmental and Physical Disabilities*, 14, 19–35; Coleman-Martin, M., Wolf Keller, K., Cihak, D. and Irvine, K. (2005) Using computer-assisted instruction and the non-verbal reading approach to teach word identification. *Focus on Autism and Other Developmental Disabilities*, 20(2), 80–90.

40 http://inclusive.co.uk.

41 From Erikson, K. and Koppenhaver, D. (2007) *Children With Disabilities: Reading and Writing the Four-Blocks Way*. Greensboro, NC: Carson-Dellosa.

42 http://inclusive.co.uk.

43 Inclusive.co.uk

44 http://oxfordowl.co.uk offer an extensive range of free e-books from the *Oxford Reading Tree* range.

45 See http://lindamoodbell.com for information on her *Visualizing Verbalising* intervention for children who do not readily make pictures in their head, an important part of reading comprehension.

46 http://inclusive.co.uk.

47 Ibid.

48 Ibid.

49 Topic sheets will be discussed later in the chapter.

50 Brown, E. (2006) *Handa's Surprise*. London: Walker Books.

51 Erikson, K. and Koppenhaver, D. (2007) *Children With Disabilities: Reading and Writing the Four-Blocks Way*. Greensboro, NC: Carson-Dellosa, p. 136.

52 http://tarheelreader.org.

53 http://books4all.org.uk.

54 In *Clicker 7*, from the *Quick Start* page, got to *Files* tab in the top left of the screen, then *Learning Grids* on the bar on the left. You can search by curriculum area, or the type of resource you want, e.g. Clicker book or Word Bank.

55 http://splash-city.com.

56 http://inspiration.com/kidspiration.

57 Available on the Mac App Store. See http://attainmentcompany.com for more information.

58 Anderson, K., Balandin, S. and Clendon, S. (2011) He cares about me and I care about him. Children's experiences of friendship with peers who use AAC. *Augmentative and Alternative Communication*, 27(2), 77–90.

59 Stanton, M. (2014) *Can I Tell You about Cerebral Palsy? A Guide for Friends, Family and Professionals*. London: Jessica Kingsley.

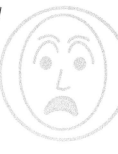

60 Justdifferent.org

61 http://disabilityactionalliance.org.uk.

62 http://legislation.gov.uk.

63 See Chapter 16.

64 http://legislation.gov.uk. *Equality Act* (2010).

65 See Chapter 16.

66 Anderson, K., Balandin, S. and Clendon, S. (2011) He cares about me and I care about him. Children's experiences of friendship with peers who use AAC. *Augmentative and Alternative Communication*, 27(2), 77–90.

67 Kate Caryer is a writer, actor and founding member of the Unspoken Project, CIC. See http://theunspokenprojectcic.com/about. Kate Caryer has won awards for her contributions to the Arts and was the first continuity announcer using AAC on Channel 4.

68 Toby Hewson is co-chair of Communication Matters and is Company Director of http://justdifferent.org.

69 Martin Pistorius is author of the bestseller autobiography *Ghost Boy*, about his experiences of discovering AAC.

70 http://nspcc.org.uk/globalassets/documents/schools/underwear-rule-pants-presentation.pdf.

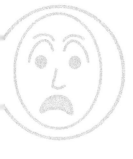

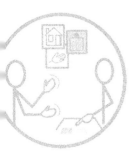

Chapter 13

Widening horizons

Secondary school and further education

The transition to secondary is a huge one. Secondary school presents new challenges, which include:

- The physical environment is bigger, requiring movement between multiple learning environments. AAC equipment, including accessories and mounting will need to travel too.

- The sensory experiences are different, with a range of environments including busy cafeterias and corridors. Children with physical, sensory or social communication difficulties may feel vulnerable or stressed at these times.

- There is a sudden jump to independent learning. There is an expectation that students will organise their own equipment, be aware of the timetable, complete work in a timely manner, and carry out some of their own research for learning tasks.

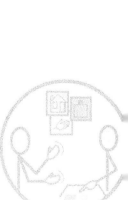

- At primary school, the AAC user may have been known by all staff and students. They would have had a limited number of teachers in a day. At secondary school, the AAC user must interact with multiple new teachers and peers who are unfamiliar with their AAC systems.

Transition planning

Transition planning takes time, ideally an academic year ahead. It should consider all areas of learning needs and the demands of the new secondary school day. Teaching and therapy staff from both settings should meet before the transition to put together a plan for:

- Practicalities of transport to and from school, toileting, medications, eating and drinking, and moving equipment around the school.

- Training new staff in positioning and moving and handling the student safely.

- Training new staff in therapy interventions, including physiotherapy, or management of eating and drinking.

- Training new staff in the use of AAC systems, including Aided Language Stimulation and communication partner training, and using the specialist hardware and software. This may be done over a few sessions.

- Steps that may be taken to increase a student's access to the school environment and the educational and social activities on offer. This may include environmental adaptations, and a child's access to computing facilities.

- Steps that may be taken to make the AAC user feel secure and safe in the new environment. A buddy or mentoring system may be put in place. There may be a supportive environment that the AAC user can access when they are tired or stressed.

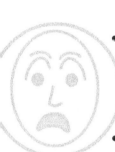

- Visual supports may be used by teaching staff to support the AAC user, or be adopted generally by the school. These should include a communication passport (see next section) and a visual timetable for the student.

- Discussion about how to ensure high-quality teaching across the school: how to motivate and engage this student; strategies to aid their understanding and increase their participation, and ways to make resources accessible.

- Adaptations that may be made to the timetable, in order to accommodate therapy activities, or to allow catch-up time to complete written work using the student's alternative written recording method.

Communication passports

These are helpful in managing transition. They can take many forms. At a most basic level, they might have brief information about how the student communicates and what to do to help. They may be extended to include information on the student's physical and sensory needs, medical information and emergency contacts. Information about the software that the student uses can be useful, as unfamiliar teaching staff may be unaware of the potential applications, and this may whet

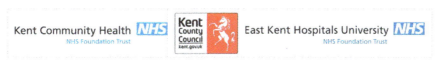

Kent and Medway Communication and Assistive Technology Service (KM

My Communication Passport

How I communicate…

I use a little Makaton signing, facial expressions, my PODD communication book and a Voice Output Communication Aid (VOCA).

Insert Photo Here

I am Ines

My VOCA is an iPad mini .
I access my VOCA using the index finger on my right hand. I am encouraged to wear my hand splints. I use the Compass Communication software .

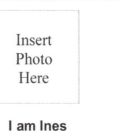

Communication Book

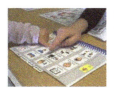

This needs to be available for when I cannot use my VOCA for example when I am driving my wheelchair or in the bathroom.
It is important that I can let you know how I feel and what I want to do at all times.
Please use **yes** and **no** symbol cards to make sure you understand my choices.

Widgit Symbols (c) Widgit Software 2002-2016   www.widgit.com

Figure 13.1 My passport

A communication passport as a booklet[1]

their appetite to find out more. Screenshots are recommended, to make the passport attractive and user-friendly. The student should be involved in designing the communication passport, so that they are happy to use it. The communication passport may be a booklet if there is lots of information to convey, or could be as subtle as a credit card.

Support for Written Recording Across the Curriculum

I can use a regular laptop or computer but I need to have access to my joystick and switch on the Maxess tray.

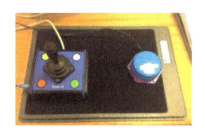

I can use a computer for my written recording. I use Clicker 6 **matching grids**, **sentence building grids** and other activity grids to complete activities in many subjects.

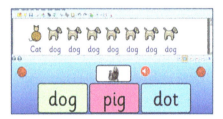

Clicker 7 and computer set up

- I need the computer to be positioned so that the top of the screen is level with my eyes.

- I use a larger mouse pointer which can be downloaded from the **Ace Centre** (see attached sheet)

- I need to be reassured that it is okay to make a mistake but I can complete my work with encouragement. **Don't let me give up too easily!**

Widgit Symbols (c) Widgit Software 2002-2016   www.widgit.com

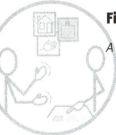

Figure 13.2 Support

A communication passport as a booklet[2]

Equipment Set Up

VOCA set up

- Please turn my VOCA on when I come in the classroom and make sure it is fully charged at the start of each day.
- I need my VOCA placed on my tray, table or fixed to the bracket on the mounting pole attached to my wheelchair so that I can reach it without leaning or stretching
- Please check that I can see the screen clearly and that light is not reflecting on it and it is cleaned with screen cleaners.
- You may need to move it to one side when I am completing written recording on the computer using my joystick and switch but I still need to be able to talk **so please remember my VOCA is my voice.**
- I need to have access to my VOCA throughout the day in order to make requests, answer questions in class, join in group discussions and make social comments.
- You may need to personalise my VOCA from time to time and add new vocabulary. Please ask the Speech and Language Team in school.
- My VOCA may occasionally need updates so that it continues to work efficiently.

If you have a technical problem that you cannot resolve with the VOCA please contact the KM CAT service on 01233 629859

If you have a technical problem that you cannot resolve with the VOCA please contact ....

Widgit Symbols (c) Widgit Software 2002-2016   www.widgit.com

Tips for Success

Please be patient...
It takes me time to settle. Please give me time to think and prepare what I want to say.

Model to me...
You can use my VOCA to talk with me and show me how to say something. I need to see you using it so I can learn where the words are.

Remember...
My VOCA might go wrong. Please remember the other ways I can communicate, such as my Communication Book, Makaton signing and Yes and No symbol cards and help me to use these

I want to join in...
Expect me to take part in everything and give me a chance and encourage me to communicate for a variety of reasons.

I may need help...
I need you to get my VOCA out as soon as I arrive and make sure it is fully charged ready for a busy day. Any problems please tell the speech and language team as soon as possible.

I need working breaks...
I will need to do this every few minutes to help me, it is very difficult for me to concentrate for long periods of time. give me short tasks to complete followed by a relaxation break.. I work

I am easily distracted by noise and movement and what other people are doing please show me what to do a couple of times and make sure the tasks are short and clear.is the best way to help me work.

Widgit Symbols (c) Widgit Software 2002-2016   www.widgit.com

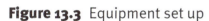

Figure 13.3 Equipment set up

A communication passport as a booklet[3]

Independent learning

No teenager wants a Teaching Assistant (TA) permanently attached to their side. The role of any support staff will need to be discussed and agreed on during the transition process. Rather than being with the AAC user all the time, a TA may spend some of their time preparing resources for lessons. TAs need to have time built into their schedules for meeting with teachers to plan adaptations. It is important that teachers make topic vocabulary available before the start of term so that this can be added to the AAC device or made into a topic vocabulary sheet.[4] Lesson plans may also be shared. It is preferable that a number of staff members are competent in using the student's AAC system, so that there is contingency planning for staff absence or change. The role of the TA will vary for each AAC user, but may include:

- Transporting and setting up AAC equipment at the start and end of each lesson.

- Programming relevant curriculum vocabulary onto the device or making topic vocabulary sheets.

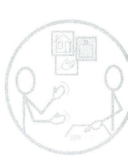

- Preparing curriculum software resources, or downloading pre-made curriculum resources (e.g. *Clicker* word banks and learning grids[5] or *WriteOnline* word bars and writing frames).[6]

- Scribing a student's quick ideas for planning work.

- Taking screenshots or printing work and storing these in a way that allows the student to access them. There will need to be a filing system, by subject. These screenshots and printouts may also be collated, along with videos and photos, as evidence of the student's normal way of working for exam access (see below).

- Creating visual supports or apps to help the student to organise their work (e.g. homework planner, timetable, revision schedule, mind-maps).

- Accessing online resources. *Books for All*[7] is a website created by CALL Scotland offering a wealth of alternative format books, including many textbooks and revision guides. Whilst these are designed for Scottish qualifications, many are relevant to the curriculum in England, Wales and Northern Ireland.

- Adding learning outcomes for each lesson to the AAC system to help the student retain information for the next lesson, and for revision purposes.

- Advocating for the AAC user where learning situations could be improved or where physical or social access could be improved.

- Promoting social interaction with peers (e.g. sharing communication strategies; withdrawing where appropriate to give the AAC user privacy and autonomy).

- Adding relevant words and phrases to the "Chat" page, based on those used by peers. Peers may help with this, as they will have a better understanding of street talk!

- Assisting with personal care.

- Monitoring progress towards outcomes and working with the teaching staff and Special Educational Needs Coordinator (SENCO) to make appropriate changes to the provision.

- Informing relevant therapy staff of any changes in need with regard to positioning, access or AAC system.

Curriculum software and recording

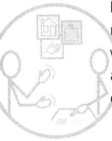

In the last chapter we explored curriculum software like *ChooseIt!* and *Clicker*. These may still be appropriate for the secondary student. *ChooseIt!* and *SwitchIt!*, along with many other primary resources, will continue to be relevant for students who attend special school provision. The most useful software or types of software are outlined in Table 13.1.

Table 13.1 Software

Software	Key Features	Educational Uses
Clicker[8]	• Text-to-speech for reading and editing work. • Word banks of important vocabulary. • Word prediction to enhance rate of typing. • Insert pictures and audio easily. • Writing frames for a range of genres. • Thousands of pre-made activities available online.	Word processing and producing multimedia documents for all subjects, including mind-maps, posters and booklets. Compatible apps for iPad are available.
Write Online[9]	• Text-to-speech for reading and editing work. • Word bars (equivalent to word banks in *Clicker*) of important vocabulary. • Word bars could include academic language, e.g. modern languages and scientific terms. • Word prediction to enhance rate of typing. • Insert images easily. • Writing frames for a range of genres, including essays. • Sentence-starters for essay-writing. • Website links for more information can be in inserted into writing frames.	Word processing and producing documents for all subjects, including mind-maps, posters and booklets. It is a more adult version of *Clicker*, which will be suitable for further and higher education, and work. Windows and Mac versions. Compatible app for iPad is available. Requires a good internet connection in all parts of the school. Suitable for higher education too.

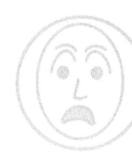

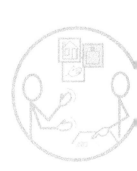

(Continued)

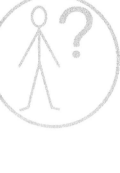

Table 13.1 (Continued)

Software	Key Features	Educational Uses
	• Workspace for planning work or revision. • Thousands of online resources available. • Range of access options, including switch-scanning. • High-contrast settings for visual impairment. This software is currently being updated and will be released with a new name shortly. See http://cricksoft.com for details.	
Penfriend[10]	• Text-to-speech for reading and editing work. • Screen magnification. • Specialist lexicons (similar to word banks in *Clicker*) can be imported, including modern foreign languages and scientific terms. • Word prediction to enhance rate of typing. • Speaks phonemes. • Dictionary and thesaurus. • Integrates with *Clicker* for switch accessibility.	Word processing for all subjects. Not as versatile as *Write Online* or *Clicker*, but is compatible with *Clicker*, and word processing may be all a specific user needs. Portable version comes on a USB stick, which can be used with a wide range of hardware. Suitable for higher education too.

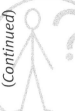

(Continued)

Software	Key Features	Educational Uses
Read&Write Gold[11]	• Text-to-speech for reading and editing work. • Compatible with a range of web browsers, so that website material can also be accessed using text-to-speech. • Picture dictionary. • Talking calculator. • Images and text from websites can be stored in "fact folders" and used in documents.	Word processing for all subjects. Research for all subjects. Onscreen talking calculator for maths. Compatible with a range of web browsers. Windows and Mac versions available. Suitable for higher education and work.
Co:Writer[12]	• Text-to-speech for reading and editing work. • Word prediction uses the context of the sentence, and has all possible spelling patterns including personal patterns. • Simple interface on screen. • University edition is available.	Word processing for all subjects. Research for all subjects. Compatible with a range of web browsers. Compatible with all computer applications, including social media and email. Compatible with Windows and Mac. Suitable for higher education and work.
Splash![13]	• Maths activities and drawing tools for making charts, graphs and diagrams, including geometry activities. • Science resources are also available, e.g. labelling diagrams for biology, drawing chemistry apparatus and physics models.	Written recording for maths and science subjects. Not fully switch-accessible yet, but likely to be developed.

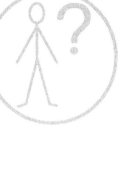

Table 13.1 (Continued)

Software	Key Features	Educational Uses
Geogebra[14]	• Maths software for geometry, graphs, algebra, statistics, spreadsheets and calculus.	Suitable for GCSE and A Level Maths, and for higher education. Compatible with Windows, Mac and Linux.
MathType[15]	• Mathematical notations and equations can be generated and used in a range of documents.	Suitable for GCSE and A Level Maths, and for higher education.
chemdoodle[16]	• Drawings for scientific experiments. • Diagrams to show biochemical structures, e.g. cells, carbohydrates.	Suitable for GCSE and A Level Biology, Chemistry and Physics, and for higher education.
Grapevine[17]	• Allows alternative access to all Windows applications on a PC, laptop or tablet. • A range of onscreen keyboards with a "stay on top" feature, full mouse functions with direct or indirect access. • Text-to-speech for all applications. • Allows web browsing, access to social media and the creation of a variety of documents.	Research for all subjects. Access to all computer applications. Suitable for GCSE, A Levels and higher education.

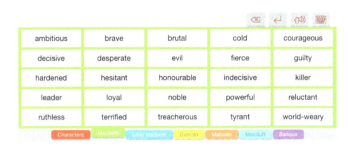

Figure 13.4 Write Online

Write Online *word bars for discussing Shakespeare's* Macbeth

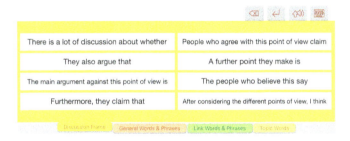

Figure 13.5 Write Online 2

A Write Online *writing frame, with essay sentence-starters.*

The range of software may seem overwhelming. Schools and therapists are advised to consult their local and regional AAC Services for advice before purchasing software for an individual. Suppliers can also offer advice and training.

It is crucial that curriculum and recording software is in place early on in the student's secondary career to prepare for exams (see the section 'Exam Access'). It is recommended that schools seek support from Year 7 to ensure that the student is using the most appropriate software for their needs. Hub and Spoke AAC services will be able to advise (see Chapter 10).

Street-talk and text-talk

An important aspect of a young people's identity is the language they use. It is important that AAC users have access to this. The most appropriate phrases will be different for every individual. It may be a useful project to work with an AAC user and a group of supportive peers to select a suitable vocabulary for chatting. Street-talk dictionaries for different parts of the UK are available online. Be prepared for hilarity or humiliation as young people inform you that you are hopelessly out of date. These are a starting point, and can be refined. They will need to be updated as the young person progresses through secondary school, as an AAC user in the sixth-form will want different phrases to those they had in Year 7.

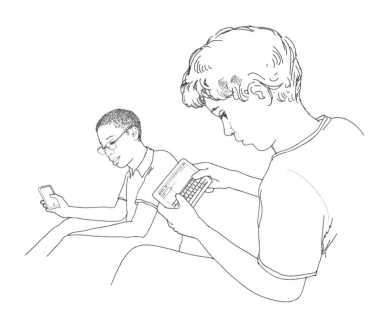

Balancing AAC with speech

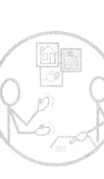

For AAC users who have little or no functional speech, this issue is likely to have been addressed earlier in their development. However, for some AAC users, there may have been enough functional speech for there to be hope that this will become their main mode of communication. Secondary school is often a time when speech sound work is reviewed. If there has been little or no progress, then the Speech and Language Therapist should discuss this with the young person and their family. Therapy may focus instead on compensatory strategies, including the use of AAC, and communication repair strategies.

Some individuals with unclear speech who use AAC as a backup have limited insight into their own communicative effectiveness, and so do not make use of their AAC as much as would be optimal.[18] This may be exacerbated by communication partners being unwilling to indicate when they have not understood. Social communication groups such as *Talkabout*[19] may be helpful in addressing this sensitively. Hustad and Shapley[20] advocate that AAC users are taught the skills to identify communication breakdown and strategies to resolve difficulties.

Interestingly, research suggests that an AAC user's family are often more reluctant to use and value AAC as an alternative to speech than the AAC user themselves.[21] This may be because parents hold on to a hope that the young person will speak, whereas the young person experiences more success (at least outside of the home) with AAC.[22]

Because families can often use prior knowledge and contextual clues to work out their child's speech, they are often unaware that outside the home, their child is not understood. If families are given this information in a sensitive manner, they can see the need for AAC to support speech, and the focus of Speech and Language Therapy intervention may move away from speech sound work and on to using AAC in combination with verbal and non-verbal communication, and communication breakdown repair strategies.

Internet safety

This is an issue for all young people, and adults need to be informed in order to help young people manage risk. AAC users may have internet access on their device in order to access other applications such as a web browser, email or social media.

The NSPCC produce up-to-date guidance for all children and young people on their website.[23] Advice includes:

- Have conversations early and often about internet safety. Explain the risks in language the child understands. You might talk about "bad" or "mean" people and "scary" videos with a young person with developmental delay. Present the internet as a fun place, but with dangers. Have a page on the child's AAC system where you can talk about online activity, with the capacity to build phrases, so that the child can talk about their experiences and report issues.

- Explore online together, so that you are informed about your child's activity.

- Know who your child is talking to online. Make sure that they have a parent or other trusted adult as a "friend" to monitor activity on social media sites. Young people with developmental delays and social communication difficulties are especially vulnerable, so consider delaying their access to social media, or monitoring more closely.

- Set boundaries around online activity: how much, which sites, what to share, and being respectful (never say anything you wouldn't be prepared to wear on a T-shirt). Create a visual support to use before online activity, to remind the young person about the rules.

- Make sure that content is appropriate. Stick to age-ratings for games. A disturbing image or video cannot be erased once it has been seen, so be proactive in avoiding exposure to inappropriate content.

- Use internet filters and parent controls. K9[24] is free and is easy to use. Our service installs K9 on all AAC devices that are to be used by children and young people.

- Check privacy settings in apps and games. Use the strictest settings, and review them regularly.

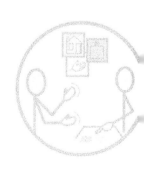

- Talk about what to do if your child sees something upsetting or experiences cyberbullying.

- If your child breaks the rules you have set, then consider using "Guided Access",[25] whereby you lock them in to specific apps (e.g. communication apps) so that they cannot access the other functions of the iPad or tablet. Different operating systems have different ways of doing this.

Young people with developmental delay and/or social communication difficulties may be especially vulnerable online, as they are less able to judge appropriacy. They are likely to need extra support in managing online activity. Working in a social skills group might be one way of monitoring and revisiting online safety on a regular basis. A consistent message between home and school is also important, so this should be agreed.

Identity development and AAC

Adolescence is a time when young people start to forge their own identity. They become more aware of similarities and differences, and how they fit in, or don't fit in, with society's norms. An individual's sense of identity is influenced by their gender identification; sexual orientation; racial, ethnic and cultural identification; religion, nationality and regionality; sub-culture; interests and abilities. A young person may become more aware of their disability at this age. Adolescents typically do not like being different, and they may be sensitive to having AAC equipment that makes them stand out. AAC may be more accepted if it incorporates important aspects of the young person's identity. The chat page might include favourite bands or TV programmes, and topics that are really important to that individual. There might be links in the vocabulary package to favourite websites (e.g. sports or music news). The AAC hardware might reflect the young person's personal aesthetic (e.g. with the homescreen or case).

Social inclusion

Every individual plays various social roles at different times in their life (e.g. son/ daughter, brother/sister, student, friend, girlfriend/boyfriend, volunteer, worker, member of a group). Social connectedness contributes to our sense of wellbeing, and ultimately, mental health. How willing a young person is to use their AAC in different situations will depend on their own motivation, attitude towards AAC, confidence in giving it a go, and resilience in the face of failure.[26] Those working with the young person can help establish what might help or hinder social inclusion, but here are a few ideas:

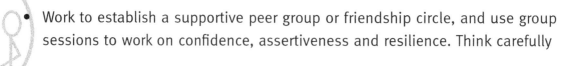

- Work to establish a supportive peer group or friendship circle, and use group sessions to work on confidence, assertiveness and resilience. Think carefully about the selection criteria for the group. Establish and maintain ground rules so that the group is safe.

- Explore a range of media in the group, as a vehicle for sharing thoughts and feelings. For example, pieces of music, works of art, poems, news articles.

- Provide the young person with the vocabulary and phrases that enable the exchange of ideas around topics that are important to them. During adolescence, music often becomes important. Or it may be gaming, films, sports or TV.

- Incorporate positive feedback at the end of each session (e.g. one thing you said that I thought was interesting).

- Provide teaching of social communication skills such as initiating and terminating a conversation, maintaining the topic, taking turns in a conversation and assertiveness skills. Programmes like *Talkabout*[27] address these issues.

- Devise an introductory phrase that the AAC user could use with new people (e.g. "I can understand what you say, but need time to program my talker. I can say yes by looking up and no by looking to the side").

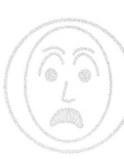

- Similarly, phrases for putting new communication partners at their ease. For example "it's OK, I know this feels a bit weird . . ." This will have to suit the personality of the AAC user.

- Encourage the AAC user to ask other people questions, and to use conversation maintaining phrases, like "really?" "that's interesting", or "that's funny".

- Incorporate the sort of language that peers are using (e.g. "LOL" and "hashtag"). Swear-words are important too. An AAC user has to learn to regulate their use of these, just like any other young person.

- Provide strategies for repairing communication breakdowns, and for coping with vocabulary not being available. A page with phrases like "it's similar to . . .", "it's the opposite of . . .", "it sounds like . . ." can be useful for this. Also phrases like "that's not quite what I meant", and "I'll try to say it in a different way."

- Enable the AAC user time to interact with peers without the presence of teaching staff. It may be necessary to carry out preliminary work, like gauging group dynamics, the group's awareness of difference, the communication and AAC skills of peers, and their ability to repair communication breakdown.

- Consider having a mentor in school for the AAC user. This may or may not be another AAC user. Choice of mentor will be crucial, and the AAC user should have input into this, and be involved in evaluating the usefulness of such a project.

- Janice Light carried out research into an internet-based mentoring programme,[28] which matched adult AAC users with young people. The mentors and protégés were able to discuss issues around education, relationships, family, transport communication and technology. Ninety-six per cent of mentors and protégés reported satisfaction with the programme. It may be a role of voluntary organisations such as Communication Matters or Regional AAC Hubs to set up similar programmes in the UK.

- Provide opportunities for meaningful group projects. This is a common way that students extend their friendship networks in school. The purpose of the project should be related to an interest of the AAC user. For example, it might be around developing an art installation or a music performance. Or it may be part of the curriculum.

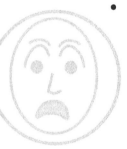

- Incorporate discussions about diversity into the PSHE (Personal Social Health and Economic) curriculum.[29] There may be a focus day on AAC, using positive role models and guest AAC speakers. Make sure that the AAC user is comfortable with this. *Just Different*[30] is an organisation providing workshops for schools to promote social inclusion. They work to the PSHE curriculum requirements for all key stages.

Conversation partners

It might be time to revisit Aided Language Stimulation, but with more of a focus on social inclusion. Peers might be trained as conversation partners, possibly using video feedback to enhance their skills (see Chapter 14 for a more detailed description of such a training programme).[31]

Any training will have to be sensitively implemented, with consultation with the AAC user, the school and Hub and Spoke AAC services. Some training is better than no training, and so even a brief awareness session using the "10 Top Tips" in Chapter 14 will be better than nothing.

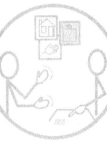

Speech and Language Therapists are often skilled in the use of video feedback to enhance communication partners' skills.[32] Short videos of interaction can be used to identify helpful strategies that partners are using, and to reflect on why that is helping. This positive slant is important: noticing the positive elements reinforces them, and results in increased use. Noticing negative elements damages the partner's confidence, and makes them less likely to engage. The person themselves may notice negative elements, and the facilitator might ask them to reflect on what they could do instead, and why that might help. The AAC user might be included in the training too. Possible strategies to notice are:

- Being positioned where you can make eye contact;

- Giving the other person an opportunity to initiate conversation;

- Responding to the other person's turn;

- Showing interest in what the other person is saying;

- Waiting for the AAC user to formulate their message;

- Checking the meaning of the message where needed (e.g. if it is a comment or question);

- Helping to clarify the message where needed;

- Using a balance of comments and questions;

- Encouraging the use of alternative strategies (e.g. onscreen keyboard, semantic clues page);

- Using multi-modal communication where needed.

If video consent and the practicalities of videoing prove difficult, then these strategies may be discussed in a group, and there may be opportunities for practise and review without the use of video. To engage peers in conversation partner training, this might be offered as the "new skills" component of the Duke of Edinburgh Scheme.[33]

Environmental barriers and supports

Environmental barriers and supports[34] may hinder or help the AAC user to reach communicative competence. Environmental barriers or supports can come from policies or practices that are in place (e.g. transport, timetabling), from the attitudes of others (low expectations, resistance to technology), or the knowledge and skills of others (knowledge of AAC and supportive strategies). When discussing how things are going with a young person, it is helpful to consider the barriers that are preventing social inclusion, and supports that might be put into place, to allow functional change.

Exam access

Exam access is currently one of the biggest policy barriers encountered by AAC users. We have seen in Chapter 12 how curriculum software such as *Clicker* can allow a young person to demonstrate their ability, bypassing the obstacles of visual processing, fine motor skills and motor-planning. It may be abundantly clear that

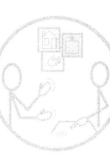

a young person needs their AAC and assistive technology to show their learning. However it is often still not possible for young people to use these technologies to access exams. Knowledge barriers mean that technologies such as using word banks or spelling prediction in word processing are mistakenly thought of as cheating.

Scotland is currently leading the way in digital exam access. The Scottish Qualifications Authority (SQA) provides electronic exam papers for AAC users. In 2015, there were 3,540 requests for digital papers for 1,487 candidates. Electronic papers are sent securely to the school, and can then be set up on a computer or iPad. The student enters their answer onto the device. Courses and webinars are provided by CALL Scotland, and there is an excellent website[35] providing information.

The following text is taken from the Joint Council for Qualifications (JCQ)'s[36] webpage about access arrangements for exams.

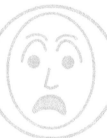

Reasonable adjustments

- The Equality Act Chapter 2010 requires an Awarding Body to make reasonable adjustments where a disabled person would be at a substantial disadvantage in undertaking an assessment.

- A reasonable adjustment for a particular person may be unique to that individual and may not be included in the list of available Access Arrangements.

- How reasonable the adjustment is will depend on a number of factors including the needs of the disabled candidate/learner. An adjustment may not be considered reasonable if it involves unreasonable costs, timeframes or affects the security or integrity of the assessment.

- There is no duty on the Awarding Bodies to make any adjustment to the assessment objectives being tested in an assessment.

The website indicates that for 90% of online access applications regarding a student with SEND, there will be an instant automated decision. For more complex cases (most AAC users), applications will be forwarded to the relevant awarding body. Schools and colleges must allow sufficient time for this process. This is generally 4–5 months before the exam. For qualifications with a coursework component, the school must apply before the start of the course. Schools therefore need to be well-informed about these arrangements!

Schools must submit information about the students "normal way of working" and provide evidence that this has been in place for a length of time. It is ideal if schools have evidence dating back to Year 7. Even though the specific software may have been updated as the student has progressed through school, the use of alternative access, text-to-speech, word banks or word prediction is likely to have been consistent. The "normal way of working" might include:

- Use of communication charts, books, and topic vocabulary charts.

- Use of visual supports (e.g. writing frame).

- Use of specialist hardware, such as a VOCA. VOCA messages may be transcribed by a TA, or screenshots or printouts taken as evidence of learning.

- Use of an alternative mouse or switch-scanning.

- Use of eye-gaze software.

- Use of specialist communication software, such as a symbol- or text-based communication package, including onscreen keyboard with word prediction.

- Use of specialist curriculum software for word processing, with word prediction and word banks.

- Use of specialist software for presenting work visually (e.g. graphs and charts for maths; mind-maps, presentations, posters or booklets for any subject).

- Use of specialist software for web browsing.

- Extra time for completing work. Alternatively, key skills may be "cherry-picked": they may be assessed once, without the student needing to repeat the same skills several times in the same assessment.

- Advanced word-prediction software, such as that used in communication packages and curriculum software like *Clicker* and *Write Online* can enhance a user's typing rate by as much as 58%. There is increased cognitive load in using word prediction, as the user has to assess which of the suggested words, if any, are appropriate. However, this is offset by the increased rate of output. The rate enhancement of word-prediction software is the difference between a student being able to sit an exam in one session, or needing to sit it over several sessions. This is the student's normal way of working and they demonstrate their understanding of the subject by constructing a meaningful sentence. They still demonstrate understanding of the subject because they have to select the right word.

If a child is to use their AAC system in exams, then the relevant curriculum vocabulary should be added and used through the course of their studies, to

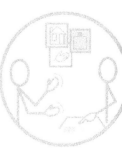

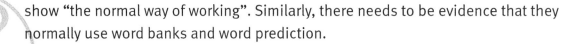

show "the normal way of working". Similarly, there needs to be evidence that they normally use word banks and word prediction.

The Joint Council for Qualifications (JCQ) website gives examples of access arrangements which may be allowed, provided that this is the student's normal way of working. There is a lack of detail about AAC, and so I have produced Table 13.2 which gives possible AAC examples. The JCQ adaptation examples in the left-hand column are taken verbatim from the JCQ website. I have added what I feel to be appropriate AAC-specific adaptations for AAC users in the right-hand column. These will be individual to the AAC user, so not all adaptations will be made. These must reflect the student's normal way of working.

Table 13.2 JCQ

JCQ Adaptation Example	AAC-Specific Adaption
Adaptation of assessment materials	• Electronic exam papers and answer sheets. • Text-to-speech software to read the paper. • Appropriate font size and colour contrasts for students with visual impairments and visual processing difficulties.
Adaptation of the physical environment for access purposes	• Accessible for wheelchair users. • Appropriate seating and positioning. • Reduced visual or auditory distractions. • Examination to take place in a separate room to other candidates if voice output is being used.
Adaptation to equipment	• Low-tech AAC, e.g. communication book, topic vocabulary charts. • Specialist computer hardware, e.g. laptop, VOCA. • Alternative access, e.g. alternative mice, switches, eye-gaze. • Mounting of AAC and computer equipment.
Assessment material in an enlarged format or Braille	• Electronic exam papers. • *SuperKeys* software for typing.

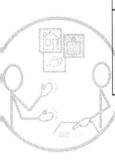

JCQ Adaptation Example	AAC-Specific Adaption
Assessment material on coloured paper or in audio format	• Including in electronic form. • Text-to-speech software.
British Sign Language (BSL)	• Symbolised text (SymbolStix, PCS, WLS) if this is the student's normal way of working.
Changing or adapting the assessment method	• Use of a VOCA with screenshots or printouts, or with a scribe. • Use of specialist software for word processing, including use of word prediction and word banks. • Alternative documents that show proof of learning, e.g. mind-maps, presentations, booklets for coursework.
Changing usual assessment arrangements	• Cherry-picking key areas to be assessed where extra time is not workable, e.g. where student would need a threefold increase in time to complete the work, and the exam is already 2 hours.
Extra time, e.g. assignment extensions	• This will depend on how the AAC user's working rate compares with their peers.
Language modified assessment material	• Symbolised text, if this is the student's normal way of working. • If vocabulary is not available on the student's VOCA, then they might paraphrase or use alternative wording in their answer.
Practical Assistant	• To ensure correct positioning of AAC equipment. • To set up eye-gaze, communication and curriculum software. • To turn pages or manipulate examination materials. • To scribe VOCA messages.
Prompter	• To remind the AAC user of all the modes available to them: low- or high-tech. • To notice fatigue and to take appropriate action.

(Continued)

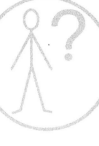

Table 13.2 (Continued)

JCQ Adaptation Example	AAC-Specific Adaption
Providing assistance during assessment	• For personal care. • For AAC, e.g. partner-assisted scanning.
Reader	• Use of text-to-speech software.
Scribe	• To scribe VOCA messages.
Use of assistive software	• Eye-gaze • Switch-scanning • Alternative mice • Symbol- or text-based communication package • Curriculum or word-processing software, including word banks and word prediction.
Use of assistive technology	Specialist curriculum software for: • Drawing graphs, charts or diagrams in Maths, Science or Geography • Producing mind-maps, presentations and booklets in English, History and Social Sciences • Producing visual media in Art and Design or audio-visual work in Music.
Use of CCTV	• To prove that the work is that of the student, and not prompted by a TA or technology.
Coloured overlays, low vision aids	• Including for electronic versions.
Use of a different assessment location	• Where the assessment will take much longer and will require regular breaks. This may be in the student's home.
Use of ICT/responses using electronic devices	• Light-tech AAC • High-tech AAC, i.e. VOCA • Text-to-speech software for checking work • Word-prediction software for word processing • Word banks for word processing.

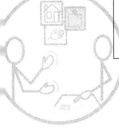

The JCQ website notes that "not all of these adjustments will be considered reasonable, permissible or practical. The learner may not be allowed the same adjustments in all exams".

Because of the lack of detail of the access arrangements in relation to AAC on the JCQ website, these aspects are worth highlighting with the exam board.

- Word processing is allowed, but with the grammar and spelling checker disabled. This suggests that word prediction software is not generally allowed. If the student has a scribe, they cannot generally gain the 5% of marks that are typically available for SPAG (spelling, punctuation and grammar). Word prediction software may be agreed to be performing the same function, and therefore the 5% of SPAG marks will not be awarded.

- There is no reference in the guidelines or in the examples to word banks. The provision of word banks is giving an AAC user access to vocabulary which may be interpreted as prompting. However the AAC user then has to put the vocabulary into meaningful sentences to answer a question, thus demonstrating the relevant knowledge. Discussion with the exam board is recommended. In most cases, word prediction will be the solution.

This process is onerous and time-consuming. I would expect exam boards to liaise and agree protocol to reduce the workload for individual students. At present the process may put schools off from entering AAC users for exams. However if we are not entering able AAC users for GCSEs and A levels, then we are severely limiting (preventing) their access to higher education and the enhanced work opportunities. Therefore, I would urge schools to put in place the following safeguards:

- Early assessment for AAC and AT to enable students to use appropriate hardware and software, and so that this is their "normal way of working". Liaise with Local and Hub AAC Services for the best solutions. Communication Matters has a forum for AAC professionals to seek advice and share experiences.

- Implementation of advice, with time for problem-solving and fine-tuning of the AAC or AT solution.

- Provide evidence to the exam board that this is "the normal way of working" for this student. Print their work, take screenshots of the curriculum software

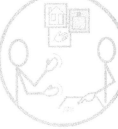

and vocabulary package, take photos of their access and mounting, enclose reports and advice from the Local and Hub AAC Services.

- Provide contact details and/or written submissions by these Local and/or Hub AAC Services.

- Speak to exam boards directly to provide additional explanation.

- Appeal if necessary. Refer to the Equality Act 2010.[37] If you know that this student has a similar level of ability to their peers, but that access is limiting their ability to show their knowledge, then you need to fight their corner.

SQA is a member of JCQ. I would urge JCQ to draw on the experience of SQA, and encourage all members of the JCQ to follow their example in providing easy-to-access information and support to secondary schools, to enable electronic exam papers to be widely used by AAC users.

Advocacy: engaging the young person in their intervention plan

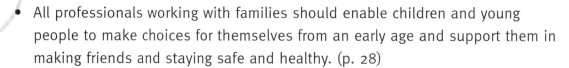

The Code of Practice[38] sets out clear expectations about the involvement of the young person in planning intervention and support. For example:

- All professionals working with families should enable children and young people to make choices for themselves from an early age and support them in making friends and staying safe and healthy. (p. 28)

- As children grow older, and from Year 9 in school at the latest, preparing for adult life should be an explicit element of conversations with children and their families as the young person moves into and through post-16 education. (p. 28)

- The provision of information, advice and support should help to promote independence and self-advocacy for children, young people and parents. (p. 32)

- As a child reaches the end of compulsory school age (the end of the academic year in which they turn 16), some rights to participate in decision-making about Education, Health and Care Plans (EHCP) transfer from the parent to the young person, subject to their capacity to do so, as set out in the Mental Capacity Act 2005. (p. 32)

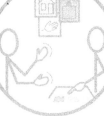

The range of available study programmes post-16 is broad and includes AS- and A-levels, vocational qualifications, apprenticeships, traineeships, supported internships and bespoke packages of learning. Careers advice should be sought. The young person should also be thinking about independent living in the future. Measures should be taken so that the young person's view is heard and noted. The following are suggestions to enable such discussions to take place.

- The young person needs to be able to make an informed choice about their options for post-16 education. It will help to visit educational settings and talk to staff about the options for the young person.

- For able AAC users, the use of visual thinking tools like mind-maps may help in making decisions. For example, if the choice is between studying for A Levels or a vocational qualification, this involves consideration of many factors.

- Opinion charts such as *Talking Mats*[39] are a valuable tool in advocacy in establishing likes and dislikes for leisure activities and programmes of study.

- Information needs to be presented in an accessible format. If information is presented in a symbolised form, then read it back without looking at the text to check that it makes sense. Don't symbolise every word, just the key words that are important for conveying meaning.

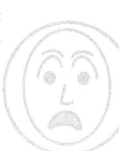

- This is a good time to review the AAC user's core vocabulary and their ability to use this functionally. This includes the ability to say that something is wrong.

- Consider the social inclusion of the AAC user. Having a variety of meaningful social roles protects against future mental health issues such as depression and anxiety.

- Consider the health needs of the AAC user. Plan for them taking more responsibility managing their needs and appointments.

- Independence skills for transport are another important consideration. Make sure that the AAC user has relevant vocabulary, and consider the use of a communication passport.

- Adult language will need to be added to the young person's AAC system. They need to have access to vocabulary that includes words for sexual activity, preferences and relationships.

- Language around safeguarding and reporting concerns also needs to be added to the AAC system.

- Plan well ahead for the transition from school into further and higher education.

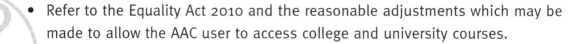

- Refer to the Equality Act 2010 and the reasonable adjustments which may be made to allow the AAC user to access college and university courses.

As discussed earlier, there may be barriers to an AAC user accessing further and higher education. For example, a young person with disabilities may need to have a reduced timetable due to health needs and fatigue. The Code of Practice states:

> **When commissioning provision, local authorities should have regard to how young people learn and the additional time and support they may need to undertake coursework and homework as well as time to socialise with their college peers within the college environment. In some cases, courses normally offered over three days may need to be spread over four or five days where that is likely to lead to better outcomes.[40]**

It is the role of those professionals working with the AAC user to clearly state their learning needs, and if necessary to advocate for reasonable adjustments to be made.

Secondary School: The AAC Toolkit

- Provide a communication passport.
- Provide basic communication partner training.
- Provide Aided Language Stimulation, unless the AAC user has reached language competence.
- Encourage multi-modal communication.
- Provide low-tech AAC, including a basic communication chart, alphabet and number chart. These could be combined on a double-sided chart.
- Consider positioning, access and mounting.
- Provide appropriate curriculum software.
- Work closely with the Hub and/or Spoke AAC Service to monitor and adapt low-, light- and high-tech AAC solutions.
- Provide for social inclusion and independence.
- Provide career guidance to plan for the future.
- Plan early for access to exams.
- Encourage independent thinking around future aspirations.
- Plan well ahead for transition to adult services.

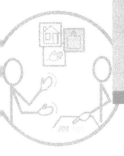

Notes

1 This template has been designed by Christine Cotterill and Hester Mackay at Kent and Medway CAT Service.

2 This template has been designed by Christine Cotterill and Hester Mackay at Kent and Medway CAT Service.

3 This template has been designed by Christine Cotterill and Hester Mackay at Kent and Medway CAT Service.

4 See Chapter 12.

5 http://cricksoft.com/uk/products/clicker and http://learninggrids.com/uk.

6 http://cricksoft.com/uk/products/writeonline. See Chapter 6 for more information about curriculum software.

7 http://books4all.org.uk.

8 http://cricksoft.com/uk/products/clicker.

9 http://cricksoft.com/uk/products/writeonline.

10 http://penfriend.biz.

11 http://enablingtechnology.com/texthelp-read-and-write-gold-115–208-p.asp.

12 http://inclusive.co.uk.

13 http://splash-city.com.

14 http://geogebra.org.

15 http://dessci.com/en/products/mathtype.

16 http://chemdoodle.com.

17 http://inclusive.co.uk.

18 Hustad, K. and Shapley, K. (2003) AAC and natural speech in individuals with developmental disabilities. In Light, J., Beukelman, D. and Reichle, J. (eds.), *Communicative Competence for Individuals Who Use AAC: From Research to Effective Practice*. Baltimore: Paul H. Brookes, p. 54.

19 Kelly, A. (2009) *Talkabout for Teenagers: Developing Social Communication Skills*. Speechmark.

20 Hustad, K. and Shapley, K. (2003) AAC and natural speech in individuals with developmental disabilities. In Light, J., Beukelman, D. and Reichle, J. (eds.), *Communicative Competence for Individuals Who Use AAC: From Research to Effective Practice*. Baltimore: Paul H. Brookes, p. 55.

21 Culp, D. and Carlisle, M. (1988) *PACT: Partners in Augmentative Communication Training*. Tucson, AZ: Communication Skills Builders.

22 Hustad, K. and Shapley, K. (2003) AAC and natural speech in individuals with developmental disabilities. In Light, J., Beukelman, D. and Reichle, J. (eds.), *Communicative Competence for Individuals Who Use AAC: From Research to Effective Practice*. Baltimore: Paul H. Brookes, p. 58.

23 http://nspcc.org.uk.

24 http://1.k9webprotection.com.

25 For iPads and iPhones.

26 Light, J. (2003) Shattering the silence: Development of communicative competence by individuals who use AAC. In Light, J., Beukelman, D. and Reichle, J. (eds.), *Communicative Competence for Individuals Who Use AAC: From Research to Effective Practice*. Baltimore: Paul H. Brookes, pp. 13–25.

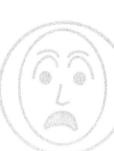

27 Kelly, A. (2009) *Talkabout for Teenagers: Developing Social Communication Skills*. Speechmark.

28 Light, J., McNaughton, D., Krezman, C., Williams, M., Gulens, M., Currall, J., Galskoy, A., Herman, M. and Cohen, K. (2000) *The Mentor Project: Sharing the Knowledge of AAC Users*. Mini seminar presented at the biennial conference of the International Society for Augmentative and Alternative Communication (ISAAC), Washington, D.C.

29 http://pshe-association.org.uk.

30 http://justdifferent.org/how-does-a-workshop-help-your-school/.

31 For a model of conversation partner training, see Kent-Walsh, J. and McNaughton, D. (2009) Communication partner instruction in AAC: Present practices and future directions. *Augmentative and Alternative Communication*, 21(3), 195–204.

32 Cummins, K. and Hulme, S. (1997, Autumn) Video: A reflective tool. *Speech and Language Therapy in Practice*, 4–7.

33 http://dofe.org/skills.

34 Light, J. (2003) Shattering the silence: Development of communicative competence by individuals who use AAC. In Light, J., Beukelman, D. and Reichle, J. (eds.), *Communicative Competence for Individuals Who Use AAC: From Research to Effective Practice*. Baltimore: Paul H. Brookes, pp. 25–32.

35 http://adapteddigitalexams.org.uk.

36 http://jcq.org.uk. The Joint Council for Qualifications is a body representing the seven main exam boards in the UK. This includes GCSE and A Levels, as well as vocational, technical and functional skills qualifications.

37 http://legislation.gov.uk.

38 Department of Education (2015) *Special Educational Needs and Disability Code of Practice: 0 to 25 Years*.

39 http://talkingmats.com.

40 Department of Education (2015) *Special Educational Needs and Disability Code of Practice: 0 to 25 Years*, p. 133.

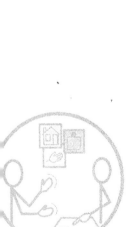

Chapter 14

Into the world of university, work and independent living

As we saw in Chapter 3, the AAC population is diverse, and so there will be wide variations in peoples' aspirations for education, work, independent living and social participation.

Transition into adult services

We need to prepare AAC users for the choices ahead of them as they move from children's and young people's services into adult services. This is a good time to review AAC systems, and the AAC user's competence in relation to Light's four AAC communicative competencies (see Chapter 17). Transition planning should be in place well ahead of time to allow the team around the young person to work on short-term goals which contribute to the long-term outcomes and aspirations.

Some considerations for AAC in this transition process are:

- Would a communication passport be useful? In nearly all cases, the answer will be "yes". See Chapter 13 for information about communication passports.

- Who will take responsibility for the long-term planning and management of AAC competency? AAC users with an Education Health Care Plan (EHCP) will continue to have at least annual reviews, and their AAC systems should be integral to this. If there is no EHCP in place, there should be another process for monitoring AAC.

- Who will take responsibility for the maintenance of AAC systems? This may include charging the device, updating software, backing up the software and adding new vocabulary.

- Who does the AAC user and key people contact in case of faults with the AAC system? Similarly if a device needs replacing, who will carry out the reassessment (Hub or Spoke AAC Service)? This will depend on the complexity of the AAC user's needs.

- What new vocabulary might the AAC user need in their new academic, work and social roles? This is likely to continue to evolve throughout adulthood, depending on new opportunities, interests and experiences. This might include vocabulary and phrases around:

- Specialist academic language for formal study

- Technical language for an apprenticeship or job

- Hobbies and interests

- Current affairs and topics that are trending on social media

- Intimate relationships, including sexual and emotional needs

- Accessing public transport and ordering from cafés and shops

- Independent living arrangements

- Recruiting personal assistants

- Financial planning and budgeting

- Medical and therapy appointments

- Managing health needs, including diet, exercise and sexual health

- Managing wellbeing and mental health

- Reporting concerns, abuse or crime[1]

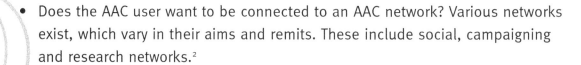

- Does the AAC user want to be connected to an AAC network? Various networks exist, which vary in their aims and remits. These include social, campaigning and research networks.[2]

Further education

This includes sixth-form colleges, further education (FE) colleges, 16–19 academies and independent specialist colleges. A wide variety of programmes of study are available, which may include formal qualifications like A Levels, vocational training, or preparation for independent living. The Code of Practice[3] emphasises high aspirations for young people with SEN. Where higher education is not under consideration, then work-based learning is recommended. This may include:

- Apprenticeships: paid jobs that incorporate training, leading to a professional qualification.

- Traineeships: education and training programmes with work experience. These last for a maximum of 6 months.

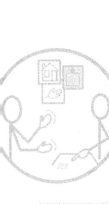

- Supported internships: unpaid job experience of at least 6 months, with support to move on to paid work.

Access to work funding (see "The Workplace" later in this chapter) is available for these programmes. Young people with SENs should receive careers advice at school to prepare for the most appropriate route. The Code of Practice suggests "job-carving": tailoring a job so that it is suitable for a particular worker and their skills. Local authorities should provide supported employment services to match students to suitable workplaces, and this is included in the Local Offer (see Chapter 16).

The Code of Practice[4] also states that where young people have EHCPs, local authorities should provide a full package of education, health and care provision for young people across five days a week, which may include non-educational activities such as:

- Volunteering or community participation

- Work experience

- Independent living and travel training

- Training in maintaining friendships and support in the community.

Higher education

Universities, colleges and institutes of technology and vocational schools come under the umbrella of higher education. For brevity in this section, I will refer to "university". University should be the aspiration for AAC users who are academically able. Careers advice should have been provided at secondary school from at least Year 9 to allow planning for this.

Where an EHCP is in place, the local authority should plan a smooth transition to higher education before ceasing the EHCP. They should plan how social care support will be maintained, and whether this will take place in the home local authority or the area they are moving to. Once a young person's place at university has been confirmed, the local authority must pass a copy of the EHCP to the relevant person at university at the earliest opportunity. Tuition fees for higher education for young people with EHCPs are paid for by the Education Funding Agency (EFA) and local authority.

Universities, like schools, are obliged to make "reasonable adjustments" to comply with the Equality Act 2010.[5] The same rules apply, whether the student attends university on campus or through distance learning. Each university has a Disability Support Service.[6] In larger universities there will be a team, with representatives in each school, and a designated officer for each student. Their responsibilities include:

- Managing the transition to university with the student and their family. The practicalities of accommodation, transport, car parking and emergency procedures will be high on the list initially.

- Pastoral care to manage personal issues associated with the transition to independent living and study at university, including mental and physical health and wellbeing. The Disability Support Service can link students with the University Occupational Health and Counselling Service as needed.

- Training for university staff, including lecturers and tutors, so that course materials are accessible. This will also include training for library and IT staff, so that they can effectively support a student in their studies.

- Physical accessibility to facilities at university, including lecture theatres, tutorials, libraries, labs and social spaces. Some equipment may require modification (e.g. to make lab equipment accessible).

- Assistive technology appropriate to the course of study. This may include digital recorders for lectures or magnifiers for paper resources. It also includes specialist software, access and mounting. Advice should be sought where necessary from Hub or Spoke AAC Services, AAC organisations and suppliers where more bespoke high-tech solutions are needed. These organisations may also be able to offer support and training.

- Timetabling flexibility. There is generally more flexibility in higher education, as part-time and distance learning are well-established options. Depending on the course of study, there may be greater blocks of time for independent study. Some students may need help in organising their time effectively. Regular personal tutorials may help in addressing difficulties.

- Library accessibility with e-books and e-journals. There is variability in the actual accessibility of these, depending on the platform being used.[7] The platform should allow "magnification with reflow" so that a complete line of text is visible. The platform should also have "recolour" options, so that the text and background colour can be altered. There should be text-to-speech reading by page or by highlighted area. DAISY digital talking books are now widely used. These synchronise audio output with highlighted text, and offer easy navigation. Changes in copyright law mean that accessible copies of texts can be made and shared between institutions. See http://cilip.org.uk and http://altformat.org for more information on this.

- Study skills support to help students with their organisation, academic writing, research skills, revision strategies and exam technique. This can be specific to the challenges for an AAC user.

- Exam arrangements that are personal to the student. This will include assistive technology, extra time, breaks and so on.

- Social inclusion. There are myriad social groups and societies at university, offering scope for new social roles. There is typically a disability rights presence at university, which may be a novel experience for AAC users.

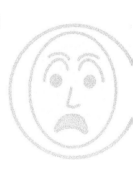

- Students with disabilities may be more vulnerable to radicalisation, being taken advantage of, or criminal activity, and so work around safeguarding and reporting within the university is vital.

- Student life is traditionally hedonistic, which may be problematic for students with disabilities who have complex health issues to manage. Sexual health, alcohol and drug awareness, personal safety and mental health are all issues that Students' Unions can offer support with, in conjunction with Disability Support Services.

- Advice about finances.

Disabled students are eligible for the Disability Students' Allowance (DSA).[8] A student can claim this if they study part-time, as long as they study at least 25% or over of a full-time course. The DSA covers four areas:

- Specialist equipment allowance, including assistive technology such as a computer or laptop, specialist software, access and mounting.

- Non-medical helper allowance, including note-takers or specialist study skill support. This would include setting up AAC and AT.

- General disabled students' allowance, including costs of photocopying, IT access and insurance.

- Reasonable spending on travel costs.

The student may also receive Disabled Living Allowance (DLA) to help with personal care.

The workplace

Workplaces are also required to comply with the Equality Act 2010 in order to make reasonable adjustments. An employer should ask whether a job applicant requires any reasonable adjustments, or "access requirements" for any part of the recruitment process, to ensure that disabled applicants can participate in the process to the best of their ability. An AAC user may request that interview questions are provided ahead of the interview, to enable them to program their responses. This is different from asking about health-related questions, which the employer is not permitted to ask about before making a job offer. Once a job offer has been made, the employer can ask about reasonable adjustments that may be made to enable to candidate to carry out their duties. These adjustments include:

- Do changes need to be made to how things are done? For example, flexible working, reduced hours.

- Are physical changes to the workplace necessary? For example, rearrangement of furniture, ramps.

- Is additional equipment needed? For example, assistive technology like specialist software, alternative access or mounting.

A government scheme, Access to Work, can help with advice and costs for employers.[9] Larger organisations are likely to have an Occupational Health Team to assist with recommendations for changes and provision of equipment.

The AAC user should be aware of employment law and the Equality Act 2010. This covers recruitment, pay and conditions, sickness absence, promotion, training, dismissal and redundancy. It may be helpful to join a relevant trade union, all of which have disability teams.

Ability[10] is a magazine about assistive technology at work. It includes editorial comment and articles about new developments and current political issues around supporting AAC and AT users. The British Assistive Technology Association (BATA)[11] also provides up-to-date information about assistive technology in the workplace.

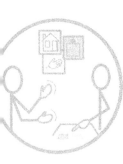

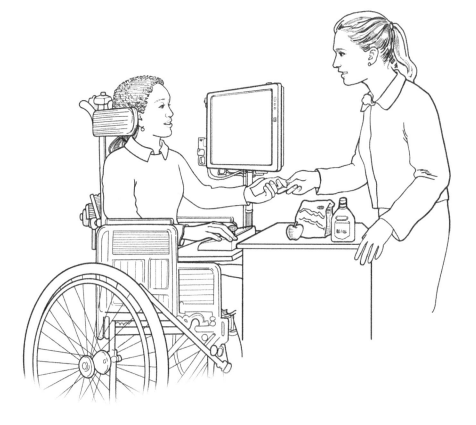

Learning disabilities, advocacy and care plans

Adults with Learning Disabilities and Autism Spectrum Condition (ASC) who have a mental health condition or behaviour which challenges should have a person-centred care and support plan.[12] The individual should have input into this, so that they are able to make choices about how their health and social care needs are met, where they live, and purposeful activities. At key points in their lives, individuals should have access to independent advocacy. There are some useful advocacy resources for adults who use AAC or have disabilities. One such resource is *Communicate With Me* by Goodwin, Miller and Edwards.[13] *The Big Book of Blob Feelings*[14] is another useful resource, as are *Talking Mats*. The individual's AAC system may need to have appropriate vocabulary added to reflect the options available.

Communication partners[15]

Communication partners include family and close friends, peers and colleagues, people in the community, and professionals who meet the health, education or social care needs of the individual. These people will have varying degrees of familiarity with AAC and how to communicate with the AAC user. Some degree of communication partner training is recommended when an AAC solution is provided for an individual. It is important to work with the AAC user to identify who they would like to receive training. Training may take the form of an AAC Hub or Spoke Professional giving advice and support, providing written guidelines, providing structured video feedback, or offering regular group support.

Kent-Walsh and McNaughton[16] identified four areas for communication partner instruction:

- Leaving more pause time, or expectant waiting

- Being responsive to communication attempts

- Use of open-ended questions

- Modelling use of AAC system.

There is therefore considerable overlap here with Aided Language Stimulation (see Chapter 9), but with less of a focus on language modelling. Kent-Walsh and McNaughton found that various training programmes for AAC users and their communication partners led to significant gains. Communication partners became less dominating in conversation and provided more communication opportunities for the AAC user. The AAC users initiated more, took more conversation turns, showed increased conversational reciprocity and used a wider range of communicative functions.

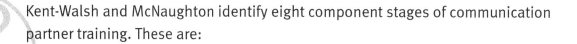

Kent-Walsh and McNaughton identify eight component stages of communication partner training. These are:

1 Pre-test and commitment to the training.

2 Strategy description: the trainers explain what the strategy is, and its importance. A way of remembering the strategy may be explored.

3 Strategy demonstration: the trainers show the strategy and examine the component skills and steps. The trainer will think aloud, talking through the how and why of what they are doing, including problem-solving and self-cueing.

4 Verbal practice of strategy steps: the trainees verbalise the steps in using the strategy.

5 Controlled practice and feedback: in a structured situation, with gradual fading of trainer feedback.

6 Advanced practice and feedback: in multiple real-life environments, with gradual fading of trainer feedback.

7 Post-test and commitment to long-term use: review of skills with the trainee in comparison to the pre-test baseline. Reflection on its impact, and action plan for generalisation and maintenance of the skills.

8 Generalisation of targeted strategy use: long-term plan for using strategy in everyday situations.

This same sequence can be used regardless of the strategy being targeted. It can be used with the AAC user themselves, as well as communication partners.

For less frequent communication partners, it may be useful for the AAC user to have a communication passport (see Chapter 13), with top tips for communication partners. These are shown below.

10 Top Tips for New Communication Partners

- Make eye contact, and interact at eye level if possible.
- Introduce yourself.
- Talk directly to the AAC user.
- Check with the AAC user how they indicate "yes" and "no".
- Ask the AAC user to demonstrate how they use their AAC.

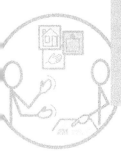

- Give the AAC user plenty of time. It's OK to be silent whilst they are using their AAC.
- Don't finish the AAC user's message unless they give you permission.
- Don't ask too many yes/no questions. Ask open questions, or offer comments, and wait for the AAC user to do the same.
- Pay close attention to the AAC user's facial expressions and body language in case there is misunderstanding. Check that you have understood the message correctly.
- Be honest if you don't understand. Ask the AAC user if they can say it in a different way. Seek assistance from a familiar partner if the AAC user gives permission.

Adult safeguarding

We must talk to AAC users about keeping safe and reporting concerns. Because as a society we tend to shy away from talking openly about abuse, we can be complicit in ignoring the reality. Types of abuse include:

- Physical abuse: this includes not carrying out care-routines appropriately.

- Sexual abuse: inappropriate touching, talk or exposure to explicit materials; forcing a person to perform sexual acts.

- Emotional abuse: making someone feel worthless or incapable; coercive control and a constant threat of dire repercussions if you do not comply with demands.

- Financial abuse: controlling a person's finances or labour so that they cannot leave the abuser.

An alarming number of adult AAC users report that they have been unable to report abuse or crime because they do not have the vocabulary available to them.[17] Vocabulary highlighted as necessary includes:

- Body parts, including sexual parts of body.

- People page, including family, friends, peers and professionals.

- Verbs for different types of physical contact (e.g. "push", "pull", "touch"), for different ways of talking (e.g. "shout", "whisper") and for sexual acts (e.g. "kiss", "touch", "rape", "force").

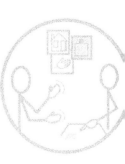

- Adjectives like "rough", "nasty", "menacing" and feelings like "uncomfortable" and "threatened".

- Phrases for reporting abuse or crime, with links to the relevant pages of vocabulary. These should be easily accessible, perhaps in the "chat page". Phrases might include: "I'm worried about . . ."; "Something happened to me"; "I need to talk to someone about abuse".

Independent Living: The AAC Toolkit

- Plan ahead for transition to adult services.

- Provide communication partner training.

- Encourage multi-modal communication.

- Provide low-tech AAC, including a basic communication chart, alphabet chart and number chart. These could be combined on a double-sided chart.

- Update AAC systems with appropriate vocabulary for their lifestyles.

- Consider positioning, access and mounting.

- Provide appropriate software for continued learning and work.

- Work closely with the Hub and/or Spoke AAC Service to develop and monitor low- and high-tech solutions.

- Provide for social inclusion and independence.

- Provide vocabulary for safeguarding.

Notes

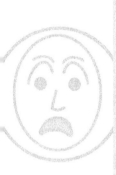

1 See the section "Adult Safeguarding".
2 Dundee University have an AAC research group for developing new AAC technologies, involving end users of software in the design and development. See http://aac.dundee.ac.uk. 1Voice is a network for AAC users and their families. It includes a team of AAC role models who successfully use AAC in their lives and act to inspire children and young people who also use AAC. See http://1voice.info. Communication Matters is the charity for AAC users, and includes a Research Involvement Network for AAC users, as well as an annual conference and roadshows. See http://communicationmatters.org.uk.
3 *Code of Practice 2014*, p. 131.
4 Ibid., p. 133.
5 http://legislation.gov.uk.

6 See http://dso.manchester.ac.uk/what-support-can-i-get for an excellent example of what a Disability Advisory Support Service can offer.

7 http://cilip.org.uk/blog/dsa-changes-short-term-purgatory-long-term-paradise? This is a really useful website from the Chartered Institute of Library and Information Professionals, who can advise on making information accessible.

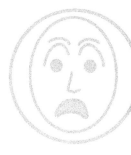

8 www.gov.uk/disabled-students-allowances-dsas.

9 www.gov.uk/access-to-work.

10 http://abilitymagazine.org.uk.

11 http://bataonline.org.

12 http://england.nhs.uk/wp-content/uploads/2015/07/ld-draft-serv-mod.pdf.

13 Goodwin, M., Miller, J. and Edwards, C. (2016) *Communicate With Me*. London: Speechmark.

14 Wilson, P and Long, I. (2008) *Big Book of Blob Feelings*. London: Speechmark.

15 For a model of conversation partner training, see Kent-Walsh, J. and McNaughton, D. (2009) Communication partner instruction in AAC: Present practices and future directions. *Augmentative and Alternative Communication*, 21(3), 195–204.

16 Kent-Walsh, J. and McNaughton, D. (2009) Communication partner instruction in AAC: Present practices and future directions. *Augmentative and Alternative Communication*, 21(3), 195–204.

17 *Alternatively Speaking*, Vol. 6, No. 3. At: http://augcominc.com/newsletters/index.cfm/newsletter_72.pdf; see http://napac.org.uk/project/was-it-really-abuse for more information about abuse and support for survivors.

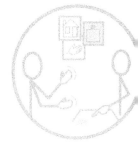

Chapter 15

Changing circumstances

The focus of this chapter is on acquired communication difficulties which necessitate the introduction of AAC. This includes stroke, head injury, changes to the structure of the head or neck due to cancer or other surgery, and degenerative conditions such as Motor Neurone Disease (MND), Multiple Sclerosis, Parkinson's Disease or Alzheimer's Disease.

Diagnosis and support

The onset and diagnosis of an acquired communication disorder is likely to be devastating for the individual and their family. It is important for health professionals to gauge the emotional needs of the person and their families, taking into consideration that people will vary in their acceptance of the situation. As with developmental disorders, there is a grief process to be negotiated. With a traumatic brain injury (TBI), there might be hope of a full recovery, which may then be modified to a partial recovery. For a degenerative condition, the grief can be ongoing, as functional abilities are affected.

The challenge of AAC

An AAC user with an acquired or degenerative condition is likely to have had typical language development and to have been a competent speaker prior to the incident or onset of disease. This can be a positive, in that we can draw on their competency.

However, there is no getting away from the fact that AAC presents a challenge and is a very different communication experience. Spoken conversation typically proceeds at rates of 150 to 250 words per minute for natural speakers who have no disabilities, whereas people who need to use AAC are typically limited to fewer than 15 words per minute.[1]

For this reason, individuals often want to make the best use of what speech they have. Speech and Language Therapy may focus on spoken language, and this is entirely valid. In the case of aphasia (the term for acquired language impairment after head injury or stroke), therapy may focus on word-finding strategies or improving sentence structure. In the case of a degenerative condition, therapy may focus on making better use of breath support for speech, or using a voice amplifier.

It is entirely valid for speech and language to be worked on alongside AAC systems in the case of head injury or stroke.[2] AAC professionals should provide information about the benefits of AAC, perhaps with the opportunity to meet other AAC users, and reassure that AAC will not interfere with the potential for speech recovery. For individuals with degenerative conditions, therapists should discuss options with the potential AAC user, being sensitive to their current preferences, but with a pathway for introducing AAC when needed.

Acceptance of AAC

Research reviews suggest that even if AAC is initially resisted, most individuals accept the need for it, once professionals have allowed them to make an informed decision. In a report by Ball et al.,[3] 96% of people with ALS (Amyotrophic Lateral Sclerosis, the most common form of MND) accepted and used AAC once it had been recommended. Ninety per cent accepted the AAC immediately. Six per cent delayed but eventually accepted the technology. In a review by Ball et al. (2004), those who rejected AAC demonstrated a co-occurring dementia or experienced multiple severe health issues, such as cancer, in addition to ALS. One hundred per cent of those with ALS used their AAC technology until within a relatively brief period (a few days to a month) prior to death, when low-technology strategies become predominant.

People with TBI are likely to need AAC for a long time, particularly if their injury was sustained whilst young. Fager et al.[4] found that 91% of this population used AAC once it had been recommended. Eighty-one per cent continued to use it after 3 years. In TBI, abandonment tended to be because of lack of facilitator training rather than the AAC user rejecting their AAC. This highlights the importance of the support of families or care providers.

Timing of AAC Support

For degenerative conditions, communication may not be the immediate priority. Mobility, physical access to work and leisure activities, and independence in feeding and personal care may be the more pressing issues early in the disease process. However, it is important that AAC is introduced in time for the user to learn how to use the system. Health professionals will need to be sensitive to the needs and preferences of the individual, and allow them to make an informed choice. It may help to see some of the AAC solutions, or to talk to an AAC professional or an AAC user ahead of time. It has to be acknowledged that the timing can be difficult where AAC users have rapidly deteriorating conditions.

It is generally suggested that clients' speech rates are monitored by the local Speech and Language Therapy Team. The frequency of checks will depend upon the

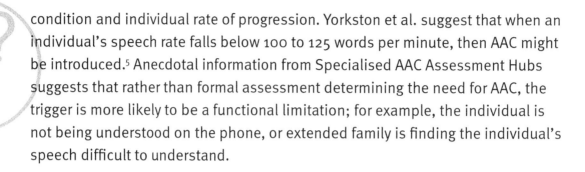

condition and individual rate of progression. Yorkston et al. suggest that when an individual's speech rate falls below 100 to 125 words per minute, then AAC might be introduced.[5] Anecdotal information from Specialised AAC Assessment Hubs suggests that rather than formal assessment determining the need for AAC, the trigger is more likely to be a functional limitation; for example, the individual is not being understood on the phone, or extended family is finding the individual's speech difficult to understand.

In addition to the slowness of AAC interaction, it also needs to be acknowledged that the nature of conversation is changed. It can be difficult for people to be spontaneous with AAC. It is difficult to interject mid-conversation with vivacity when using a synthesised voice. It is difficult to convey emotion and empathy. It is difficult to express complex, nuanced ideas. The balance of power in interaction is radically altered, with AAC users typically taking shorter and fewer turns, and being reliant on a partner to interpret ambiguous utterances.[6] There is an acknowledgement that there is often a *co-construction* of AAC messages: the communication partner will add to and clarify the AAC user's limited message, using their intuition and knowledge of the AAC user.[7] How much message completion or embellishment the partner should contribute is something that needs to be discussed and agreed with the AAC user.

AAC practitioners should acknowledge the limitations of AAC communication. It is frustrating for a competent spoken language user and their family. Negative feelings must be acknowledged and explored. Individuals often report that they struggle with the reduced eye contact in AAC communication, as both partners tend to look at the AAC rather than one another. However, if this is acknowledged, both partners might consciously check in with each other using eye contact at the beginning or end of a message.

Whilst it may be painful to discuss the prospect of not being able to communicate, it is important to be prepared for change. Adults who suddenly lose their voice report how lonely life becomes. Having some communication is better than no communication at all.

It is important to introduce resources before they are needed. AAC solutions should be introduced just in time for the changing needs of the AAC user and their interaction partners, taking into account the user's current and projected communication competencies, their physical access needs, the needs of their communication partners and the communication demands of their communication environments.

Low-tech AAC solutions

Even where high-tech AAC is the preference, a low-tech backup should also be available. High-tech AAC is not practical in the bathroom, or overnight, when a device is likely to be charged. High-tech AAC screens can be difficult to see in bright sunlight when outdoors. For degenerative conditions, towards the end of life, low-tech AAC may be more accessible than high-tech. At this time, the individual's physical needs tend to be more urgent and there may be messages that need to be quickly conveyed, without needing to set up high-tech AAC.

Commonly used low-tech AAC solutions for adults with acquired and degenerative conditions include:

- Basic communication charts (see Chapter 5). These will typically have an alphabet and numbers, and quick phrases relating to immediate and medical needs. Access may be direct or indirect via partner-assisted scanning (see Chapter 7).

- There are standard templates of basic communication charts for acute hospital settings available online.[8] These may include a pain scale, a body map, common symptoms and basic requests. They are designed for patients who have not yet been assessed for communication difficulties and are symbolised to make them as accessible as possible where literacy may be impaired.

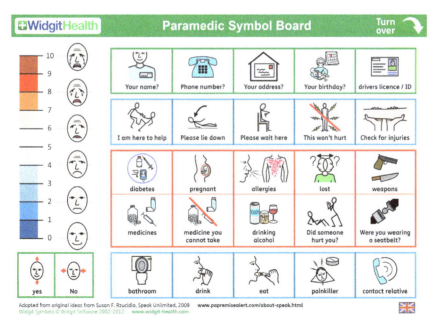

Figure 15.1 Paramedic Symbol Board.

Susan Radazzio

Widgit Symbols © Widgit Software 2002–2017 www.widgit.com

- Once a patient has been assessed by a Speech and Language Therapist, a more personalised communication chart can be developed. For about 85% of adults with acquired sudden-onset conditions, this is likely to include an alphabet chart if the user has literacy and can still use their skills. The remaining 15% of adults may use symbol or picture communication.[9]

- The Speech and Language Therapist will assess the patient's receptive and expressive language. More extensive use of visual supports will be needed if there are receptive language difficulties.

- In some cases, writing or drawing may be a suitable form of expressive communication. It may also support receptive language.

- A strategy that is of particular use to AAC users with unclear speech is to point at the first letter of a word on an alphabet chart at the same time as saying the word. This reduces the guesswork of the communication partner. Time spent with a Speech and Language Therapist will be needed to learn this skill.

- A communication passport might be used for unfamiliar communication partners (see Chapter 13). This might take the form of a booklet or a credit card.

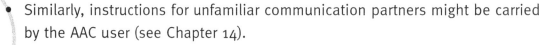

- Similarly, instructions for unfamiliar communication partners might be carried by the AAC user (see Chapter 14).

- Communication books (see Chapter 5). These should be personalised by the AAC user and their family, reflecting their preferred layout. For example, whether they are organised by topic or pragmatic function, whether they use text, symbols or photos, and whether they include biographical information or remnants. The most immediate communication needs should be placed near the front of the book.

- Photo books or low-tech Visual Scene Displays might contain contextually rich photos, which have multiple associations for the AAC user. Biographical details may be added, or phrases to stimulate extended conversations around the photograph.

- *Remnant communication books*[10] may be particularly helpful for introducing topics of conversation for those AAC users with memory or cognitive impairments. Remnants such as photos, maps, certificates, newspaper cuttings, tickets, brochures and programmes might be included. These may be used when the AAC user still has speech, or in conjunction with other AAC solutions.

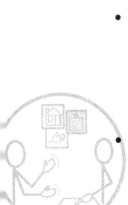

- Light-tech talking buttons may be used for getting others' attention, or for specific instructions and requests in particular places around the home.

- Other no-tech ways of getting attention may be preferred, such as raising a hand or vocalising. Just as with developmental conditions, multi-modal communication is advocated with this AAC population. Time might be spent working on strategic competence with the AAC user and their family or carers (see Chapter 17).

High-tech AAC solutions

High-tech may be more acceptable to some users, simply because it is normal to use a phone, tablet or computer. If direct access is possible, then there are relatively low-cost apps available (see Chapter 6). Text-based typing apps offer more flexibility for those AAC users who have retained their literacy skills.

Symbol-based packages are less desirable for this population of AAC users, because this is like introducing a new language. We do not want to place too many demands on cognition and memory, and so it is preferable to make use of residual language and literacy skills.

There are new innovations all the time to improve the user experience of using AAC. These are designed for the AAC user to aid with ease of using the device or software. Some of these innovations include:

- Improvement in the sound quality of synthesised speech. This is particularly important in noisy environments and where communication partners may have age-related hearing loss.[11] Bluetooth speakers are also available to pair with many communication devices.

- A range of regional accents and ages of voice are now available in synthesised speech.

- Voice-banking is an option whereby an individual with a degenerative condition can record their own voice. This needs to take place early on in the disease process, as it typically requires at least eight hours of recording. The AAC user can then use their own voice for synthesised speech.[12]

- In practice, many people with rapidly degenerating conditions choose not to undertake the process of voice-banking. Instead they choose message-banking, where specific messages are recorded using their own voice. This may include personal greetings or messages for family members (e.g. telling a partner that they love them, special sayings, or telling a favourite story for grandchildren).

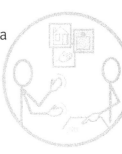

- If voice-banking of the individual's own voice is not possible, then there are other options. The MND Association is currently working with a research project in Edinburgh to build a bank of various regional accents. If there is a suitable match for an individual, then this may be used in preference to more generic synthesised voices. Voice is incredibly personal: every voice is unique, and so the AAC user needs to choose a voice that is acceptable to them.

- Word prediction software has improved in recent years, allowing individuals' spelling patterns or shortcuts to be learned. This population of AAC users is likely to make more use of spelling than those with developmental disorders.

- Spelling can be combined with quick phrases to enhance the rate of communication. Some packages learn the first letters of phrases, allowing much quicker typing (e.g. they only have to type "syla" for "see you later alligator").

- Access to quick phrases for greetings, broad topic of conversation starters, encouraging phrases, clarifying and repair phrases, and closing phrases have all been identified to be useful for the maintenance of socially appropriate conversation.[13] These can be personalised for the user.

- Communication devices such as the *Lightwriter*[14] and *Allora*[15] are commonly used with this population, making use of their literacy skills. These two devices can also be made switch-accessible, in the case of changing access needs (deterioration of function).

- Various screen layouts are available, including text- or symbol-based grids with pre-stored phrases and Visual Scene Displays. Simplified visual displays are sometimes preferred by AAC users with acquired disorders, who may find busy screens overwhelming.

- Visual Scene Displays contain contextually rich photographs that will trigger a range of associations. This may be particularly helpful for those AAC users with severe language impairments, cognitive or memory impairments. The onscreen hotspots may contain personal biographical information, and links to other pages of related content.

- Links to multimedia within a communication package may help the flow of conversation for some users.[16] The internet may be a way of introducing relevant material to stimulate conversation; for example, a link to a news website or YouTube.

- The use of mainstream computer functions and apps is particularly important for younger AAC users, who need to continue their working and social lives. These users will also have younger partners and family members who are at work or school, and so they will have a greater need for independence.

Working from home is a viable option for many more AAC users because of advances in internet technology.[17]

- Personal photos, videos or audio recordings may be added to a communication package, as a basis for communication, for example within a news page or favourites page.[18] This is important for retaining a sense of identity and social connectedness.

- A personal history may be included within a vocabulary package, to give biographical details such as education and work history, and key life events. This may also help in retaining identity. Practical details such as drug regimes and reminders might be added for users with memory problems.

- AAC users who have had a stroke or head injury are much more likely to find complicated visual displays overwhelming. Reducing the detail in visual displays and simplifying or magnifying webpages may help.

- There is increased access to mainstream apps, software, and social media, with a range of access options for computers and tablets.

- Communication software can now make use of GPS, making predictions about the phrases that might be needed in a given location. For example in a café, phrases and vocabulary for ordering a coffee will be available. It is likely that this GPS prediction will be refined in the future for topics of conversation (e.g. when the user is in an art gallery or museum, specific vocabulary and phrases relating to the exhibits may become available).[19]

- Natural Language Generation (NLG) is described by Arnott and Alm,[20] where a relatively small amount of information about an event can be programmed into the communication device (e.g. who, where, what, when), and the software converts this into coherent messages.

- RFID (radio frequency identification) tags are small devices which can be attached to objects to broadcast information about themselves to anyone nearby. Sensors are used to detect a person's presence and their interactions with objects. This technology is particularly useful for AAC users who have memory difficulties, and who might need reminders to assist with independent living.[21]

Changing access needs

The same access options that were considered in Chapter 7 are available to this population. There are some variations, including:

- Speech amplification devices may be used where there is inadequate breath support.

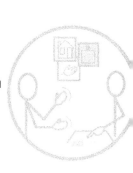

- Electrolarynxes or speaking valves may be used where there has been damage to the vocal cords.

- Speech recognition software may be used for those individuals who have some functional speech but struggle to access a computer or tablet. *Siri* for Apple devices, *Cortana* for Microsoft Windows, and *Dragon* are all examples of mainstream software. These will be less effective in noisy environments.

- Head-pointers or head-mice are often viable access methods for those with good head control. These may be preferred to eye-gaze: there is no calibration needed, users can move around more, and this method tends to be less fatiguing for the eyes.

- Alternative mice that respond to a very small range of movement (e.g. thumb mice) can be used for adults with degenerative conditions.

- Switches and switch-scanning can be used. They type of switch and its positioning will depend upon the user's range of movement.

- Infrared or electromyographic switches may be used where there is limited range of movement. These respond to the slightest of muscle movements.

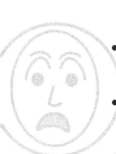

- In the case of degenerative conditions, there may be a need to change access method as physical skills change.

- Some conditions will vary from day to day, or may be relapsing-remitting, and so two different access methods may be used.

- Positioning and mounting will be of upmost importance and will require regular review for AAC users with degenerative conditions.

- Medications, fatigue and pain may all contribute to variations in functioning, and so AAC users and their facilitators need to keep AAC professionals informed of any changes.

Facilitator training

At the start of AAC intervention, it is important to identify key family members or carers who will facilitate AAC communication. This might include assistance with linguistic, social, operational or strategic competency (see Chapter 17).[22] The AAC user's needs are likely to change, some at a rapid rate, and so it is important that the identified facilitator knows that they should contact the relevant AAC professional, given certain triggers.

Beukelman et al.[23] found that primary facilitators preferred hands-on, detailed step-by-step instruction in a given AAC solution. They reported receiving slightly over 2 hours of instruction and reported that amount of training as appropriate.

In recent years a "just in time" principle has been advocated. This applies to providing the right amount of AAC support and training at the right time, and also in enabling the AAC user and their family to input into the AAC system easily, so that they can then make necessary adjustments as needed. Learning how to programme a high-tech device or add pages to a communication book allows the AAC user and their family to take ownership of the AAC system, making it more likely that it will be used. In some cases where AAC systems have been abandoned, it is the lack of facilitator support rather than the AAC user's rejection that has led to the AAC system not being used.[24]

Conversation partner training is also recommended to enhance the AAC user and their family and friends' experience of using AAC (see Chapter 14).

Changing social roles

AAC users and their families report that an acquired communication disorder or the onset of a degenerative condition leads to a huge change in social roles and participation. Social networks often shrink as functional abilities are lost. This also affects the partner or family members of the AAC user. It is recommended that family members provide some sort of information, be it verbal or written, to support less frequent communication partners. This may include ways to support mobility and physical access, as people are often uncomfortable about asking how they might help.

The physical and emotional burden on the partner of the AAC user is often the greatest. The dynamics of intimate relationships are changed. It is helpful if other family members and friends are proactive in offers of practical help and emotional support.

Support networks

As has been noted, a key part of AAC support are the family members of the AAC user. It is vital that these people get the emotional and practical support that they need. The various national charities for acquired and degenerative conditions can provide signposting and support, from counselling to respite care. Online forums or events can be further sources of information and support.

End-of-life advocacy

AAC may play an important part in helping an individual with a degenerative condition in planning for end-of-life care.[25] Studies have shown that many patients with MND wish to make advanced directives about medical interventions such as pain relief, nutrition, hydration, antibiotics, ventilation and resuscitation.[26] Preferences about where end-of-life care is to take place may also be stated (e.g. at home, in a hospital or in a hospice).

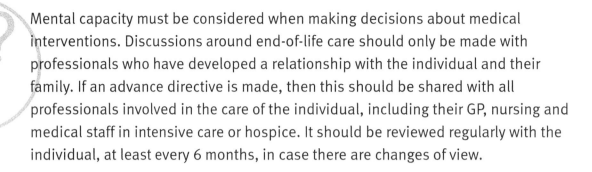

Mental capacity must be considered when making decisions about medical interventions. Discussions around end-of-life care should only be made with professionals who have developed a relationship with the individual and their family. If an advance directive is made, then this should be shared with all professionals involved in the care of the individual, including their GP, nursing and medical staff in intensive care or hospice. It should be reviewed regularly with the individual, at least every 6 months, in case there are changes of view.

Care must be taken to comply with the law and safeguarding guidelines. Support for family members should be offered, as they may be left with the guilt of either complying with their family member's wishes or being unable to do so. This may be compounded by disagreement between family members.

AAC has an important part to play in demonstrating what the individual's wishes are near the end of life. Appropriate text or symbol vocabulary, access to spelling and the ability to provide yes/no/don't know responses will be important. AAC professionals may be able to provide reassurance about the individual's capacity and communicative competence. Clear documentation must be kept. Screenshots or video may form part of this, with explanations.

A final visit from an AAC professional once an individual has died may be needed. Loan equipment may need to be collected. Whilst distressing for all, this is an opportunity for the family and professionals to have one final session to share thoughts and feelings, to offer condolences and to end what may have been a very significant relationship with the family.

Changing Circumstances: The AAC Toolkit

- Work with partner agencies to ensure timely referral.
- Provide communication partner training.
- Encourage multi-modal communication.
- Provide low-tech AAC, including a basic communication chart, alphabet chart and number chart. These could be combined on a double-sided chart.
- Consider positioning, access and mounting for changing needs.
- Provide appropriate software for continued social inclusion and quality of life.
- Provide low-tech AAC for medical emergencies and end-of-life care.

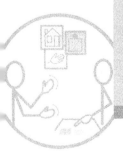

Notes

1 Beukelman, D. and Mirenda, P. (2005) *Augmentative and Alternative Communication: Supporting Children and Adults with Complex Communication Needs*. Baltimore: Paul H. Brookes.

2 Fager, S., Hux, K., Beukelman, D. and Karantounis, R. (2006). Augmentative and alternative communication use and acceptance by adults with traumatic brain injury. *Augmentative and Alternative Communication*, 22, 37–47.

3 Ball, L., Beukelman, D. and Pattee, G. (2004) Augmentative and alternative communication acceptance by persons with amyotrophic lateral sclerosis. *Augmentative and Alternative Communication*, 20, 113–123.

4 Fager, S., Hux, K., Beukelman, D. and Karantounis, R. (2006). Augmentative and alternative communication use and acceptance by adults with traumatic brain injury. *Augmentative and Alternative Communication*, 22, 37–47.

5 Ball, L., Beukelman, D. and Pattee, G. (2000) A bulbar profile prototype for assessment of individuals with progressive dysarthria. *Amyotrophic Lateral Sclerosis and Other Motor Neuron Disorders*, 1(3), 84–85; Ball, L., Beukelman, D. and Pattee, G. (2001) A protocol for identification of early bulbar signs in ALS. *Journal of Neurological Sciences*, 191, 43–53; Ball, L., Beukelman, D. and Pattee, G. (2002) Timing of speech deterioration in people with amyotrophic lateral sclerosis. *Journal of Medical Speech Language Pathology*, 10, 231–235; Yorkston, K., Beukelman, D. and Tice, R. (1996) *Sentence Intelligibility Test for Macintosh*. Lincoln, NE: Communication Disorders Software. Distributed by Tice Technology Services, Lincoln, NE.

6 McCarthy, J. and Light, J. (2005) Attitudes toward individuals who use augmentative and alternative communication: Research review. *Augmentative and Alternative Communication*, 21(1), 41–55.

7 Clark, H. H. (1996) *Using Language*. Cambridge: Cambridge University Press.

8 www.widgit-health.com/downloads/hospital-procedures.htm.

9 Fager, S., Hux, K., Beukelman, D. and Karantounis, R. (2006). Augmentative and alternative communication use and acceptance by adults with traumatic brain injury. *Augmentative and Alternative Communication*, 22, 37–47.

10 http://praacticalaac.org/strategy/communication-books-aphasia/.

11 Beukelman, D., Fager, S., Ball, L. and Dietz, A. (2007) AAC for adults with acquired neurological conditions: A review. *Augmentative and Alternative Communication*, 23, 230–242.

12 http://mndassociation.org/forprofessionals/aac-for-mnd/voice-banking.

13 Todman, J., Alm, N. and Elder, L. (1994) Computer-aided conversation: A prototype system for nonspeaking people with physical disabilities. *Applied Psycholinguistics*, 15(1), 46–73.

14 http://toby-churchill.com/products/lightwriter-sl40/.

15 http://techcess.co.uk/allora/.

16 Alm, N., Astell, A., Ellis, M., Dye, R., Gowans, G. and Campbell, J. (2004) A cognitive prosthesis and communication support for people with dementia. *Neuropsychological Rehabilitation*, 14, 117–134.

17 McNaughton, D. and Bryen, D.N. (2002) Enhancing participation in employment through AAC technologies. *Assistive Technology*, 14, 58–70.

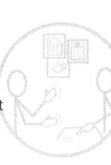

18 Alm, N., Astell, A., Ellis, M., Dye, R., Gowans, G. and Campbell, J. (2004) A cognitive prosthesis and communication support for people with dementia. *Neuropsychological Rehabilitation*, 14, 117–134.

19 Patel, R. and Radhakrishnan, R. (2007) Enhancing access to situational vocabulary by leveraging geographic context. *Assistive Technology Outcomes and Benefits*, 4(1), 99–114.

20 Arnott, L. and Alm, N. (2013, September) Towards the improvement of Augmentative and Alternative Communication through the modelling of conversation. *Computer Speech & Language*, 27(6), 1194–1211.

21 Gil, N., Hine, N., Arnott, J.L., Hanson, J., Curry, R., Amaral, T., Osipovic, D. (2007) Data visualisation and data mining technology for supporting care for older people. *Proceedings of the ACM SIGACCESS International Conference on Computers and Accessibility* (ASSETS 2007), Tempe, AZ, 15–17 October, pp. 139–146.

22 Light, J. (1989) Towards a definition of communicative competence for individuals using augmentative and alternative communication systems. *Augmentative and Alternative Communication*, 5, 137–144.

23 Beukelman, D., Fager, S., Ball, L. and Dietz, A. (2007) AAC for adults with acquired neurological conditions: A review. *Augmentative and Alternative Communication*, 23, 230–242.

24 Fager, S., Hux, K., Beukelman, D. and Karantounis, R. (2006). Augmentative and alternative communication use and acceptance by adults with traumatic brain injury. *Augmentative and Alternative Communication*, 22, 37–47.

25 Hurtig, R. and Downey, D. (2008) *Augmentative and Alternative Communication in Acute and Critical Care Settings*. Plural.

26 Borasio, G.D. and Volz, R. (2014) Advance directives. In Oliver, D., Borasio, G.D. and Johnston, W. (eds.), *Palliative Care in Amyotrophic Lateral Sclerosis: From Diagnosis to Bereavement*. Oxford: Oxford University Press.

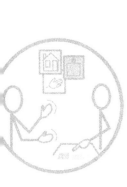

Chapter 16

EHCPs and target setting

The Code of Practice

The new Code of Practice 2015[1] reflects changes introduced in the Children and Families Act 2014.[2] These include:

- There is a stronger focus on high aspirations and improving outcomes for children and young people aged 0–25.

- There is a clearer focus on the participation of families and the child/young person (CYP) in decision-making at individual and strategic levels.

- It includes guidance on the joint planning and commissioning of services to ensure close cooperation between Education, Health and Social Care.

- It includes guidance on publishing a transparent Local Offer of services available to the CYP with Special Educational Needs or Disabilities (SEND) across Education, Health and Social Care.

- Education, Health and Care Plans (EHCP) to replace Statements and Learning Difficulty Assessments. EHCPs to cover the age range of 0–25.

- There is new guidance for education and training settings on taking a graduated approach to identifying and supporting pupils and students with Special Educational Need (SEN).

- There is a greater focus on support that enables those with SEN to succeed in their education and make a successful transition to adulthood.

- Information is provided on relevant duties under the Equality Act 2010.[3]

- Information is provided on relevant provisions of the Mental Capacity Act 2005.[4]

A graduated response to SEN

The Code of Practice sets out a graduated response to a child or young person not making expected educational progress. There should be high-quality teaching, with high levels of engagement and participation for all students in their learning, and appropriate differentiation for individuals. Where progress for an individual is less than expected, then teaching staff need to work with their Special Educational Needs Coordinator (SENCO) to assess whether a CYP has an SEN, and

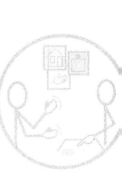

what interventions may be put in place. Broad areas of need may be identified, which are:

- Communication and interaction

- Cognition and learning

- Social emotional and mental health difficulties

- Sensory and/or physical needs.

Where a child or young person has an identified SEN, then support should be put in place, using a four-part cycle of Assess, Plan, Do, Review.[5] Where assessment indicates a need to involve specialists such as Speech and Language Therapists, this should not be delayed, and these specialists should be involved in the cycle from then on. A range of evidence-based and effective teaching approaches, appropriate equipment, strategies and interventions may be put in place to support the child's progress. There should be agreed outcomes with a review date. Where these resources have been put in place but the child or young person has not made the expected progress, then assessment for an EHCP may be requested.

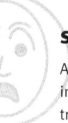

SEN and disability

A child may have a disability without having SEN. An example would be a physical impairment. A child may have SEN without having a disability (e.g. a child with a transient language delay). A child may have both a disability and SEN; examples would include many children with Cerebral Palsy, Down Syndrome, Global Delay, Autism Spectrum Condition, Specific Language Impairment and Developmental Verbal Dyspraxia. Children who use AAC all have SEN, and most have a disability.

The Local Offer

This must detail the services for children and young people aged 0–25, with and without EHCPs. This includes:

- Therapy Services, including Speech and Language Therapy, Physiotherapy, Occupational Therapy (including Spoke AAC Services), AAC and Assistive Technology Services (Hub AAC Services) and Child and Adolescent Mental Health Services (CAMHS).

- Information about different types of school provision, including mainstream and specialist provisions.

- Assessment for specialist equipment, including wheelchairs and AAC and Assistive Technology.

- How the CYP's progress will be measured.

- How professional expertise will be secured through appropriate professional development.

- Extracurricular activities, pastoral support, and social, emotional and mental health interventions.

- Information about how to request assessment for an EHCP.

The needs of some children and young people with SEND will be met by the Local Offer alone. The Equality Act (2010) sets out the legal obligations that schools and services have towards children and young people with disabilities. They must make reasonable adjustments in anticipation of a CYP attending a provision. This includes:

- Adaptations to the physical environment (e.g. reducing background noise or sensory distractions; provision of quiet spaces).

- A communication environment that supports the use of AAC.

- Flexible timetabling. This may allow for targeted and specialist interventions to take place, or may be an acknowledgement that the CYP needs more time to complete work using AAC, or that they may experience fatigue or sensory overload.

- Differentiated teaching materials. This would include the use of visual supports and symbolised teaching resources, and curriculum software like *Clicker*.[6]

- Provision of equipment. This includes items such as ear-defenders and writing slopes. It also includes no-tech, low-tech and light-tech AAC, and the use of mainstream high-tech AAC.

- Fostering of positive relationships between disabled and non-disabled children and young people.

Education, Health and Care Plans (EHCP)

Many children with SEND will have interventions in school and from specialists without needing an EHCP. There is no set threshold whereby assessment for EHCP can be instigated for a child. If support has been put in place and this is not enabling progress, then assessment for EHCP can be instigated.

An EHCP is a legal document which:

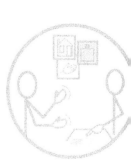

- Describes in detail the CYP's educational, health and care needs.

- Records the views and aspirations of the CYP and their parents.

- Establishes outcomes over a range of timescales and more short-term targets based on the child's needs and aspirations.

- Specifies the education, health and social care provision needed to meet the CYP's needs.

- May set out arrangements in relation to personal budgets or direct payments if this has been requested.

Embedding AAC in the EHCP

If a child uses AAC, then this needs to be specified in the EHCP. The Local Speech and Language Therapist will usually take the lead here. Communication underpins all learning. It is fundamental to the education provision. Communication and AAC is therefore an education need, rather than a health or social care need. Reference to the Child or Young Person's AAC system will however need to be made throughout the EHCP, because AAC will need to be used in all interventions. Details about the AAC systems in place will need to be updated regularly at the EHCP reviews. Table 16.1 offers suggestions for where AAC may be described within the various sections of an EHCP. Options have been included, which will need to be further specified for the individual. This suggested list of comments is not exhaustive: it is a guide only, and will need expansion. Therapists are advised to keep up to date with changes to EHCP guidelines. They should familiarize themselves with quality assurance processes locally. Recommendations should relate to the CYP's needs, and not to the services that are available locally. They should relate to what is considered good practice, for example in the RCSLT's Communicating Quality Live.[7]

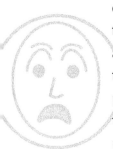

Table 16.1 Section of EHCP

Section of EHCP	Suggested AAC Detail
Section A: The views, interests and aspirations of the CYP and their parents	Provide a summary of how to communicate with CYP, and how to include them in decision-making, for example: • CYP requires spoken language to be simplified and accompanied by key word signing/symbolised visual supports. • CYP can understand 1/2/3 key words in a phrase. • CYP understands concrete language, but struggles with abstract language.

Section of EHCP	Suggested AAC Detail
	• CYP's understanding of those concepts being discussed should be checked. • CYP uses multimodal communication, which includes facial expressions/pointing/Makaton signs/yes/no response (specify this) to support their AAC. • CYP uses WLS/PCS/SymbolStix (specify) in a communication board/book/low-tech/light-tech/high-tech device (specify each). • CYP can express their views with the aid of visual supports like Talking Mats.8 Examples of aspirations might be: • CYP will achieve communicative competency using their AAC systems in a range of environments. • CYP will feel confident to join social groups or take part in social events. • CYP will have good literacy and be able to access a range of learning resources. • CYP will be able to access a further education setting or apprenticeship of their choosing. • CYP will be able to make day-to-day choices about their independent living. • CYP will manage their physical and mental health needs and understand when to seek support.
Section B: The CYP's SEN	Provide a summary of strengths and needs. A detailed description of the CYP's communication, language and speech is needed, followed by strategies to support each area of need. This should include: • Attention and listening. • Receptive language. • Expressive language. • Speech sounds. • Social communication.

(Continued)

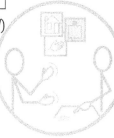

Table 16.1 (Continued)

Section of EHCP	Suggested AAC Detail
	• A detailed description of all AAC used by the child and their communication partners. • Include detailed descriptions of the no-tech, low-tech, light-tech and high-tech AAC in use. • Stress the importance of all these elements. • Aided Language Stimulation is needed throughout the day, in all environments, with all communication partners. • Cognitive levels, including processing and memory skills may fall within this section.
Section C: Health needs relating to the SEN	Medical issues such as physical and sensory impairment, epilepsy and dysphagia will need to be detailed. Advice from Physiotherapist, Occupational Therapist, Paediatrician and Dietician will be included here. • Specific AAC strategies to check the CYP's health and wellbeing may be detailed here. • Specific health pages on the CYP's AAC system can also be specified. • Because VOCAs have a shelf-life of 3–4 years, there may be a need for reassessment, support and funding for AAC equipment, including for access and mounting, from the Specialised AAC Assessment Hub and/or Local Spoke Service.
Section D: Social care needs relating to the SEN	This may include the need for short breaks, respite care, access to extracurricular and social groups. • Social communication needs and strategies can be reiterated here. • The use of AAC during these activities should be stressed. • Specific chat or social pages on the CYP's AAC system may be specified.

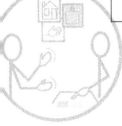

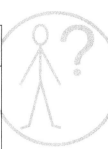

Section of EHCP	Suggested AAC Detail
Section E: The outcomes sought for the CYP	A range of outcomes over varying timescales will be developed with the CYP and their family. Outcomes might be over a key stage or school year. Targets are shorter-term steps towards the outcome, and will usually be within an academic year or term. There should be a clear distinction in the EHCP between outcomes, steps towards meeting the outcomes, provisions for meeting the outcomes, and arrangements for measuring progress. The steps towards the outcomes will be updated at least every year at annual review, and possibly more frequently. Examples of long-term outcomes might be: • CYP will use single symbols/multi-word phrases/grammatical sentences/spelling with prediction to contribute to conversations using their AAC systems by the end of the key stage. • CYP will learn the new concepts for their GCSE course and will be able to use these in Clicker grids to record their learning for coursework. • CYP will use the function buttons like home, go back, more and clear buttons on their AAC device to navigate efficiently by the end of this academic year. • CYP will be able to attempt to repair communication breakdowns, using the special page on their AAC device by the end of this key stage. • CYP will use Talking Mats or similar to contribute to the decision-making about their transition to secondary school. • CYP will be able to organise the charging of their VOCA overnight and remember to pack it in a carry case for the day's activities by the time they attend college.

(Continued)

Table 16.1 (Continued)

Section of EHCP	Suggested AAC Detail
Section F: The SEN provision	This should be specific, quantifiable and flexible. It should not be what can be provided by the Local Offer, but what the CYP needs. For example: • X hours of SLT time three times per year for joint curriculum-planning, to incorporate use of AAC, with the teacher. • X hours of SLT time for the development, creation and updating of AAC resources. • X hours of SLT time for one-to-one/small-group/within-class support each term. This may be more frequent at the start of a school term. • X hours of SLT time to provide AAC training/mentoring for school staff. • X hours of SLT time to attend the annual review and X numbers of multidisciplinary meetings to monitor the implementation of AAC in school. • X hours of SLT time for AAC planning, record-keeping, assessment, report-writing, target-setting and liaison with parents and school.
Section G: Any health provision required to meet the needs in Section C.	AAC intervention is primarily an education need, and so will not normally be part of this section. However it may be reiterated that AAC will need to be used when engaging CYP in health provision.
Section H: Social care provision to meet the needs in Section D.	AAC intervention is primarily an education need, and so will not normally be part of this section. However it may be reiterated that AAC will need to be used when engaging CYP in social care provision.
Section I: Placement	This will be completed by the Local Authority for the final plan.
Section J: Personal budget	As above.

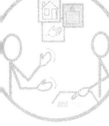

Target-setting

This section may be useful for writing the short-term steps to meet the longer-term outcomes in the EHCP.

Targets may also be set by NHS services working with adult AAC users. Various outcome measurement systems are in place in the NHS in the UK. Examples include Care Aims[10] and East Kent Outcomes System (EKOS).[11]

Towards AAC competency

If the long-term outcome is AAC competency, then we need to break this down into smaller steps.

One way of breaking this down is to look at Janice Light's AAC competencies.[12] These are:

- Linguistic

- Social

- Operational

- Strategic

In Table 16.2 that follows, I have set out some possible targets under these four competencies. Some targets have elements of more than one area of competency, but will be worded to stress the linguistic, social, operational or strategic aspect. The targets are here for inspiration, and it is intended that readers of the book will create their own targets for individual AAC users depending on current need. It is good practice to start with a baseline – what an AAC user is doing now – and to build on this baseline to make a new target. For example, the baseline for the first example might be "Katja uses the core words 'more', 'want' and 'stop' as well as other fringe words around her daily activities".

Table 16.2 Area of competency

Area of Competency	Examples of Targets
Linguistic	• Katja will learn four new core words on her communication charts and will use these in a range of play situations and everyday routines. • Katja will learn five new nouns/verbs/adjectives on the relevant pages of her AAC system, and will use these to make requests/give instructions/comment on an activity.

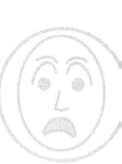

(Continued)

Table 16.2 (Continued)

Area of Competency	Examples of Targets
	• Katja will combine a noun + verb/pronoun + adjective/ adjective + noun to make a two-symbol phrase. • Katja will use three to four symbols in a phrase to talk about something she has been doing on the weekend. • Katja will use pronouns/conjunctions/verb tenses/ adverbs correctly in a sentence in formal language activities. • Katja will attempt to spell the first letter/first two letters of a word and then judge which of the four predictions is the one she needs, using her onscreen keyboard. • Katja will be able to offer four semantically related words using her VOCA when playing a guessing game with her peers. • Katja will use three new question forms on her questions page, including *when, why* and *how* in a structured activity.
Social	• Noah will sign which song he wants the group to sing at his local library sing-and-session. • Noah will direct his siblings in a game of *Simon Says*, linking two symbols, i.e. person + action. • Noah will use games phrases, e.g. "your turn", "my turn", "you won!" when playing a simple board game with one other peer. • Noah will choose which classmate will accompany him on a special job in school, using his light-tech AAC device. • Noah will join in with a class poem in their school assembly using his light-tech AAC device. • Noah will use his communication passport credit card on a trip to the swimming pool with his support worker. • Noah will use his VOCA at his respite foster placement to give opinions about activities on offer. • Noah will follow the topic of conversation, by answering a question asked by his communication partner 50% of the time in chat group.

Area of Competency	Examples of Targets
	• Noah will ask his communication partner three different questions about themselves in chat group. • Noah will recognise when it is appropriate to use swear words and adult language, and will apologise if he makes a mistake.
Operational	• Inès will activate a switch to operate a sensory toy or other device which she finds motivating. • Inès will indicate with a nod when her partner has said the desired item when using partner-assisted auditory scanning. • Inès will select cells on her VOCA using a keyguard and dibber. • Inès will use a two-step colour-coded eye-pointing to choose symbols on her E-Tran frame. • Inès will take her VOCA out of its bag and place it on the desk every morning at school. • Inès will switch her VOCA on or off at the beginning and end of the day. • Inès will toggle between her Grid 3 symbol package and Clicker 7 during class activities. • Inès will initiate calibration of her eye-gaze software when she notices that her selections are not accurate.
Strategic	• Ben will sign a word when his speech has not been understood by his communication partner. • Ben will use his communication chart at the side of his bed when his VOCA is unavailable. • Ben will add a word to his message when his communication partner prompts him for more information. • Ben will try to find a related word when he cannot find the exact word he wants on his vocabulary package.

(Continued)

Table 16.2 (Continued)

Area of Competency	Examples of Targets
	• Ben will attempt to spell a word and will use the prediction at the top of the screen to reduce the number of selections he needs to make. • Ben will use full sentences in learning situations, but will recognise that it is fine to say one or two words in a phrase when he needs to get a message across urgently, e.g. "bus here" or "need toilet". • Ben will use the quick phrases at the bottom of the page on his VOCA to start sentences. • Ben will use the grammatical function in his communication app, whereby if he presses and holds a cell, the various word endings for that word will appear. • Ben will use the alphabetical order of words in his vocabulary package to judge whether a word is on the first or second page.

Targets usually emerge from discussion with the relevant family members and professionals currently working with the AAC user. Questions to prompt ideas for new targets might include:

- What is she using well?

- What do you wish he would do more of?

- Is there vocabulary you wish you had?

- Are there phrases you wish she could say?

- In what situations is she most confident?

- In what situations is he least confident?

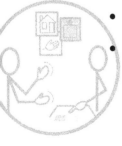

- How are you finding Aided Language Stimulation?

- Are there opportunities to use the AAC system at home/school/day centre/ respite?

- Are there more communication functions you could use? (refusing, directing, commenting, answering questions, asking questions, telling stories)

- What gets in the way of using the AAC system?

- Does she know how to use the on/off button, volume control?

- Does he use the home, go back, more and speak buttons?

- Does she navigate between pages?

- Do you know what to do when you can't find a word?

- Does he tell you when you've got something wrong?

SMART Targets

Often practitioners are required to set *SMART* targets. Definitions vary slightly, but these tend to be similar in meaning (see table 16.3).

The disadvantage of SMART targets is that they can be so specific that we can end up just training an AAC user to reach a target. The skill may be so specific that it is not generalised to other communication environments. SMART targets can take the joy out of learning, as spontaneity and creativity is lost to dull, prescriptive teaching.

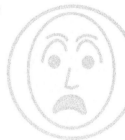

Table 16.3 SMART Targets

Specific	What the AAC user expected to do (e.g. in terms of vocabulary, syntax, pragmatics), with whom, with what resources, where, when, how often, using what communication mode.
Measurable	How will you know that the AAC user has achieved the goal? Can you count it? Can you record it?
Achievable	Given the AAC user's profile of abilities and their recent rate of progress.
Realistic	Given the resources available to support the AAC user at this time.
Time-limited	When will the target be reviewed?

An alternative to SMART targets, is SCRUFFY targets, developed by Penny Lacey.[13] These are:[14]

Table 16.4 SCRUFFY targets

Student-led	Starting from where the student is at now, but working towards a long-term outcome.
Creative	There may be several ways to meet an objective, using a variety of resources, with a number of different people and places.
Relevant	Targets need to be based on a thorough assessment of the current communication priorities, and related to the EHCP outcomes and aspirations.
Unspecified	To avoid a narrow range of opportunities and experience, and to allow for spontaneous and unexpected directions.
Fun For Youngsters	

In the table that follows, we can see how SMART and SCRUFFY targets compare.

Table 16.5 SMART/SCRUFFY

SMART Target	**SCRUFFY Target**
Anya will respond with a smile when she is presented with the light strands in the sensory room in four out of six sessions in the term.	Anya will respond to a range of visual stimuli using non-verbal communication, e.g. facial expressions, noises, in the sensory room and classroom.
Christopher will point to a food symbol from a choice of two at snack time to indicate his choice when asked by a member of staff four out of five times in a week.	Christopher will indicate his choice of activity or resource by pointing to a symbol from a choice of two during class activities such as choosing time, playtime, book-reading and singing.

Table 16.5 (Continued)

SMART Target	SCRUFFY Target
Leila will use four different verbs from the verb page in her communication book when playing *Simon Says* at home with her family. She will play the game for 10 minutes twice per week and achieve the target in 8 weeks.	Leila will use at least four different verbs from the verb page in her communication books in activities including *Simon Says*, everyday routines, looking at family photos and book-sharing. Opportunities will be provided throughout the day, and she will have achieved the target in 8 weeks.
Jakob will construct sentences consisting of Subject-Verb-Object using his high-tech communication aid in Literacy Lessons using *Language Through* Colour prompt sheets in his one-to-one time with the TA once per week.	Jakob will construct sentences consisting of Subject-Verb-Object using his high-tech communication aid and Clicker grids during one-to-one and whole-class teaching in Literacy and other lessons.

Local services will have their own guidelines and policies for writing short-term targets, and so practitioners will have to comply with these. There may be scope for using either SMART or SCRUFFY targets within an EHCP (Education, Health and Care Plan).

Notes

1 Department of Education (2015) *Special Educational Needs and Disability Code of Practice: 0 to 25 Years*.
2 http://legislation.gov.uk. *Children and Families Act* (2014).
3 http://legislation.gov.uk. *Equality Act* (2010).
4 http://legislation.gov.uk. *Mental Capacity Act* (2005).
5 *Code of Practice 2014*, pp. 101–102.
6 Clicker 7 available from http://cricksoft.com/uk.
7 See http://rcslt.org. *Communicating Quality Live*.
8 http://talkingmats.com.
9 The SLT should recommend what is reasonable for a CYP with this profile of needs, and is in line with RCSLT clinical guidelines, rather than what the SLT service can currently provide. SLTs should seek advice from more experienced colleagues as appropriate. The Local Authority will commission therapy services to provide services.

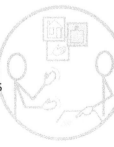

10 http://careaims.com.

11 Johnson, M. and Elias, A. (2002) *East Kent Outcome System for Speech and Language Therapy.* Eastern & Coastal Kent Community Services. (E-mail Annie.Elias@eastcoastkent.nhs.uk.)

12 Light, J. (1989) Towards a definition of communicative competence for individuals using augmentative and alternative communication systems. *Augmentative and Alternative Communication*, 5, 137–144.

13 Lacey, P. (2010, Summer) Smart and Scruffy Targets. *The SLD Experience* at http://bild.org.uk.

14 These descriptions are paraphrased from the RCSLT draft guidelines: *Guidelines for Speech and Language Therapists on their Roles and Responsibilities Under the Children and Families Act 2014 and Associated SEND Code of Practice* (2016) available on http://rcslt.org.

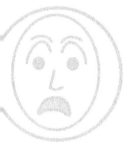

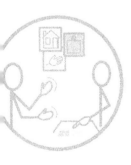

Chapter 17

AAC competencies
An overview

I am including this chapter to give a more complete overview of the AAC journey. Different AAC users will start at different points, and will progress at different rates. Some users with profound learning difficulties will work around the early targets, whilst cognitively able AAC users may whizz through these.

This section draws on Janice Light's Four AAC Communication Competencies: Linguistic, Social, Operational and Strategic.[1] The weight given to each of the four competencies will vary with the AAC user's strengths and needs, and at different stages in their AAC intervention. For example, a very young child with four-limb Cerebral Palsy may have targets in the linguistic and social areas in the early years, but would not be expected to take responsibility for the operational and strategic dimensions. A young person with Autism Spectrum Condition may focus on operational and strategic competency as they transition to Further Education. Janice Light has subsequently added psychosocial factors into her model. These include the AAC user's motivation to use their AAC system, their attitude towards AAC, their confidence in trying to use it in various situations, and their resilience in the face of failure.[2]

Because I am a Speech and Language Therapist, the linguistic competency section is very detailed! However, for a cognitively able AAC user, these steps may not need to be broken down. For example, pronouns could be worked on generally, without needing to target subject pronouns before object pronouns.

Two other assessment and tracking tools that are recommended are the Functional Communication Profile–Revised[3] and the Augmentative and Alternative Communication Profile.[4] The first one is useful for early on in the AAC assessment and intervention process, and the second is useful for subsequent intervention.

I would recommend that at any one time, a child has four short-term targets, and works on these for 3–6 months. Adult AAC users may prefer longer-term targets. Which areas of competence at any one time will depend on the AAC user. This process should be very much needs-led, and guided by discussions with the

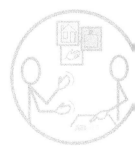

AAC user, their family and the professionals working with them. If it seems that progress is not being made, then consider a multi-disciplinary meeting to discuss ways forward. Consider a one-off consultation with the Regional AAC Hub to find solutions.

Table 17.1 Social competence

Social Competence	
Attention and Listening	• Gives fleeting attention in a "People Game", e.g. "Round and Round the Garden", "This Little Piggy". • Gives fleeting attention to a communication partner when they join exploration of a sensory toy or stimuli. • Can share attention with a communication partner for X seconds when engaging with sensory stimuli. • Can engage with a communication partner for X minutes during a motivating activity, e.g. *Attention Autism.*[5] • Can engage with a communication partner whilst playing with bubbles/ball/bricks/musical instruments/messy play.
Social Communication	• Takes a turn in exchanges of behaviour, e.g. when communication partner copies child's behaviour, the child notices. • Takes several turns in exchanges of behaviour, e.g. when partner copies child, child then does something and checks the partner's response. • Indicates pleasure during a "People Game".[6] • Uses eye contact to engage in joint play routines. • Uses non-verbal communication, e.g. facial expressions, body language, gestures and vocalisations in response to interaction. • Nods and shakes head to indicate yes and no, or has another consistent yes/no response. • Vocalises, reaches, or touches to get someone's attention. • Responds to a communication partner. • Initiates communication.

Communication Functions	• Makes a request by selecting a symbol.
	• Rejects an item or activity by selecting a "no" or "stop" symbol.
	• Comments by selecting one or more symbols on an array.
	• Answers a question by selecting one or more symbols or words.
	• Asks a question by selecting one or more symbols or words.
	• Tells a simple story about what s/he has done, using at least three symbols or words.
	• Uses symbols or text humorously, e.g. to say something that is not true and looking for a response.
	• Says how she is feeling using a symbol or text.
	• Corrects someone when they have misinterpreted a message.
	• Stays on topic with conversations.
	• Engages in conversation on a variety of subjects.
Social Participation	• Uses AAC with caregivers and siblings in a variety of play and routine situations.
	• Uses AAC to play a simple board game with a peer.
	• Uses AAC in small-group/whole-class learning.
	• Uses AAC to direct peers in an activity.
	• Uses AAC to take a message to another part of the school.
	• Uses AAC to perform in assembly.
	• Uses AAC in the community.
	• Uses AAC in extracurricular activities.
	• Uses AAC in nursery/school/college/work/Uni supportive adults in a variety of play/work/routine situations.
	• Uses AAC in nursery/school/college/work/Uni with peers.
Linguistic Competence	
Receptive Language	• Shows understanding of one key word in an instruction.[7]
	• Shows understanding of two key words in an instruction.
	• Shows understanding of three key words in an instruction.
	• Shows understanding of nouns.
	• Shows understanding of basic verbs.

(*Continued*)

Table 17.1 (Continued)

	• Shows understanding of adjectives. • Shows understanding of prepositions. • Shows understanding of six new specific verbs. • Can be assessed using formal assessments such as Reynell Language Scales, TROG or CELF.[8] • Shows understanding of a situation by appropriate expressive AAC use, using one symbol. • Shows understanding of a situation by appropriate expressive AAC use, using two symbols (and so on). • Shows understanding of a situation by appropriate expressive AAC use, using phrases containing noun, verb, adjective, etc.
Expressive Language	• Uses a single symbol to request/comment/question. • Uses four different core words[9] to request/comment/question. • Uses a range of nouns from different communication charts or different pages of a communication book. • Uses a range of verbs from the actions page of a communication book or a high-tech device. • Combines two symbols,[10] e.g. person + action, action + object, person + object, object + position, object + attribute. • Combines a core word with a fringe word. • Combines three symbols or words, e.g. person + action + object; object + position + place; action + attribute + object. • Uses a range of adjectives. • Uses basic pronouns *I, me, you.* • Uses the present progressive -ing verb ending (e.g. by selecting from the grammatical suggestions on a high-tech device).[11] • Uses the prepositions *in, on, under.*[12] • Uses plural -s. • Uses possessive -'s. • Uses articles *the* and *a.* • Uses irregular past tense for common verbs, e.g. "*fell* down". • Uses regular past tense *-ed*, e.g. "danced".

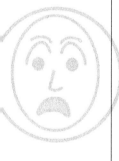

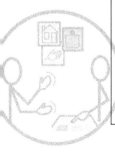

	• Uses subject pronouns *he, she, we, they*. • Uses object pronouns *him, her, us, them*. • Uses possessive pronouns *his, hers, ours, theirs*. • Uses third-person regular present tense -*s*, e.g. "eats". • Uses verb *to be* on its own, e.g. "she is happy". • Uses verb *to be* as an auxiliary verb, e.g. "she is jumping". • Uses adverbs, e.g. "quickly", "loudly". • Uses conjunctions *and, because, but*. • Uses time concepts *yesterday, tomorrow, last year, next year*. • Uses questions starting with *who, what, where*. • Uses questions starting with *when, why, how*. • Looks in relevant category page to find a word. • Uses a semantically related word when he can't find a word. • Can attempt to describe the word when he can't find it. • Uses abstract language. • Uses figurative language. • Uses academic language. • Uses technical language.
Literacy	• Attempts to spell the first letter in a word. • Spells the first two letters in a word and then chooses word from predictions. • Uses alphabet knowledge to look for a word in a page of vocabulary.
Operational Competence	
Positioning	• Is physically stable and positioned optimally for AAC access. • Recognises when AAC is not well positioned and able to use strategies to correct this.
Direct Access	• Points to symbols using a fist-point/finger-point/head-pointer/eye-point • Selects symbols using a keyguard/adapted keyboard/onscreen keyboard/stylus.

(Continued)

Table 17.1 (Continued)

	• Selects symbols using a mouse alternative (rollerball, joystick, glidepad). • Uses all the mouse functions, including right and left clicks, click and drag. • Uses eye-gaze technology for leisure. • Uses eye-gaze or head-mouse to select symbols from a grid or Visual Scene Display. • Uses eye-gaze or head-mouse to type words using an onscreen keyboard. • Uses eye-gaze or head-mouse to access curriculum software.
Indirect Access	• Indicates with a nod when her partner has reached the desired item when using partner-assisted scanning. • Uses eye-pointing with two-step colour-coding. • Activates a switch to operate a sensory toy or other device. • Activates a switch to play games on a computer or tablet. • Uses one switch with automatic scanning to make a selection. • Uses two switches to scan and select.
Operating the Device	• Can switch the device on and off. • Can put device on to charge/take it off. • Can position the device correctly. • Can indicate when something is wrong with the device set-up. • Can adjust some settings on the device, e.g. volume. • Can toggle between vocabulary package and curriculum software. • Can use different computer functions, e.g. email, social media. • Can indicate when s/he needs to change access method. • Can calibrate eye-gaze when needed.
Organisation	• Takes responsibility for carrying device. • Takes responsibility for taking the device home, charging it, bringing it to school, etc.

	• Takes responsibility for positioning device and accessories. • Edits vocabulary package. • Updates software and backs up content of device.

Strategic Competence	
Cues and Prompts	• Responds to environmental cue to use AAC. • Responds to a prompt from a communication partner to use AAC. • Spontaneously chooses AAC. • Adds more information when prompted.
Repair Strategies	• Uses the most appropriate AAC method for the situation. • Uses a different mode when one has failed. • Can choose the best access method according to position, physical state. • Tries to find a related word when s/he cannot find the exact word. • Uses the communication breakdown page to repair. • Refers partner to communication passport when necessary.
Rate enhancement	• Uses *home, go back, more* cells, or *NavBar* as appropriate. • Uses quick phrases. • Uses predictive grammar function. • Uses predictive spelling function. • Uses the most efficient navigation pathway to find vocabulary. • Uses alphabetical knowledge to find vocabulary.

Psychosocial Factors	
	• Can see the benefit in using AAC in specific communication situations (can specify which). • Wants to use AAC at home/school/college/university/work/social gatherings • Has confidence in the AAC equipment's functionality (this might be rated using a scale).

(*Continued*)

Table 17.1 (Continued)

	• Has confidence in using AAC at home/school/college/ university/work/social gatherings.
	• If communication is unsuccessful, is prepared to try again using AAC.
	• Is able to work with AAC Professionals to find solutions to functional problems with using AAC system.

Notes

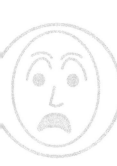

1 Light, J. (1989) Towards a definition of communicative competence for individuals using augmentative and alternative communication systems. *Augmentative and Alternative Communication*, 5, 137–144.

2 Light, J. (2003) Shattering the silence: Development of communicative competence by individuals who use AAC. In Light, J., Beukelman, D. and Reichle, J. (eds.), *Communicative Competence for Individuals Who Use AAC: From Research to Effective Practice*. Baltimore: Paul H. Brookes, pp. 13–25.

3 Kleiman, L. (2003) *Functional Communication Profile Revised (FCP-R)*. LinguiSystems.

4 Kovach, T. (2009) *Augmentative and Alternative Communication profile: A continuum of learning*. LinguiSystems. This is based on Light (1989).

5 See http://ginadavies.co.uk for more information about this fantastic intervention for developing attention in children with autism.

6 People games include games like peekaboo, tickling or swinging a child; they also involve rhymes and songs with an exciting action. The adult pauses before the exciting action and waits for a signal from the child to carry out the anticipated action. See http://hanen.org *R.O.C.K. in People Games: Building Communication in Children With ASD or Social Communication Difficulties* for more information.

7 See http://derbyshire-language-scheme.co.uk. See also http://techcess.co.uk for CARLA, a language assessment for children with physical disabilities who cannot access standard assessments.

8 See http://reynell.gl-assessment.co.uk for *New Reynell Developmental Language Scales*, http://pearsonclinical.co.uk for *Test for Reception of Grammar (TROG-2)* and http://pearsonclinical.co.uk for *CELF-Preschool 2 UK* and *CELF-5 (Clinical Evaluation of Language Fundamentals)*. These assessments tend not to be suitable for children with physical impairments, and so CARLA is an alternative (see note 7), or parts of the assessment may be used in an informal way.

9 See Chapter 5 for more information on core words. I would tend to introduce four to eight core words first, and then keep adding them as the child shows understanding and starts to use them.

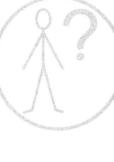

10 See Brown, R. (2013) *A First Language: The Early Stages*. Cambridge, MA: Harvard University Press for detailed descriptions of early syntax.

11 These grammatical functions will all be easier to model and learn using a high-tech device. These levels are for cognitively able AAC users.

12 Though this may be particularly challenging for children with Cerebral Palsy who have not had just extensive experience of positioning objects. Try to make this meaningful and fun, e.g. in a hiding game.

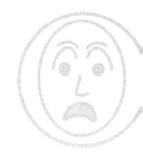

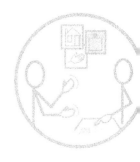

Appendix – further information

http://communicationmatters.org.uk

Communication Matters, or CM, is the UK AAC charity, affiliated with ISAAC. Communication Matters aims to increase awareness of AAC, offering education through the annual CM Conference at Leeds University in September each year, with additional Roadshows and Study Days around the UK throughout the year. There is also online training and a professional forum for members to share best practice. CM lobbies for AAC commissioning across the UK and provides up-to-date information about regional and national AAC centres in the UK. CM coordinates AAC research and provides the AAC Knowledge Research Base, http://aacknowledge. org.uk. CM is committed to AAC user involvement. The current co-chair, Toby Hewson, and patron, Martin Pistorius, both use AAC.

http://isaac-online.org

The International Society for Augmentative and Alternative Communication, or ISAAC, promotes global cooperation to share best practice in AAC around the world. There is an annual ISAAC conference at various venues each year.

http://aacscotland.org.uk

AAC resources created by CALL Scotland, an organisation commissioned by NHS Education for Scotland to raise awareness of AAC. There are downloadable resources including communication charts, posters to raise awareness, *Keep Talking* communication games, a wheel of up-to-date communication apps, and links to other AAC websites.

http://aacmanmet.wordpress.com

Manchester Metropolitan University are supported by NHS Education Scotland to provide AAC courses and resources, and to carry out AAC research. There is currently a major research project underway, led by Janice Murray, "I-ASC: Identifying appropriate symbol communication aids for children who are non-speaking: enhancing clinical decision making".

http://acecentre.org.uk

The ACE Centre is a regional AAC Assessment Hub, and provides online resources and training. There are free downloadable resources including communication charts and information booklets. The ACE Centre has developed resources to buy, including communication and curriculum software.

http://1voice.info

1Voice is an organisation for AAC users and their families. It recognises a need for a social perspective on communication and a need for adult AAC users as role models to inspire children and their families. 1Voice organises events throughout the year, with regional branches across the UK.

http://nowhearme.co.uk

A website for AAC users developed on behalf of NHS Education for Scotland, targeted at professionals in health, social care, education, and the wider world of work and leisure. There are online learning modules for those with little or no experience of AAC.

http://praacticalaac.org

PrAACtical AAC supports the international community of professionals and families supporting AAC. There is a wealth of practical resources, including videos, leaflets and posters to promote everyday AAC implementation.

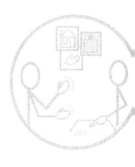